Quality Improvement in Nursing and Healthcare

A practical approach

Karen Parsley
RGN, RSCN, BSc (Hons)

Assistant Director of Nursing, Brighton Health Care Trust,
Royal Sussex County Hospital, Brighton, UK.

and

Philomena Corrigan RGN, BSc (Hons)

Clinical Nurse Advisor, Leeds General Infirmary, Leeds, UK.

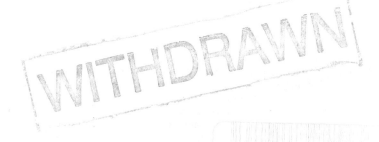

CHAPMAN & HALL

London · Glasgow · New York · Tokyo · Melbourne · Madras

Published by Chapman & Hall, 2-6 Boundary Row, London SE1 8HN, UK

Chapman & Hall, 2-6 Boundary Row, London SE1 8HN, UK

Blackie Academic & Professional, Wester Cleddens Road, Bishopbriggs, Glasgow G64 2NZ, UK

Chapman & Hall GmbH, Pappelallee 3, 69469 Weinheim, Germany

Chapman & Hall USA, One Penn Plaza, 41st Floor, New York, NY10119, USA

Chapman & Hall Japan, ITP - Japan, Kyowa Building, 3F, 2-2-1 Hirakawacho, Chiyoda-ku, Tokyo 102, Japan

Chapman & Hall Australia, Thomas Nelson Australia, 102 Dodds Street, South Melbourne, Victoria 3205, Australia

Chapman & Hall India, R. Seshadri, 32 Second Main Road, CIT East, Madras 600 035, India

Distributed in the USA and Canada by Singular Publishing Group, Inc., 4284 41st Street, San Diego, California 92105

First edition 1994
Reprinted 1995

© 1994 Chapman & Hall

Typeset in 10/12pt Palatino by Acorn Bookwork, Salisbury, Wiltshire
Printed in Great Britain by Page Bros (Norwich), Ltd

ISBN   0 412 48360 2   1 56593 236 6 (USA)

A Catalogue record for this book is available from the British Library

Library of Congress Cataloging-in-Publication Data available

∞ Printed on permanent acid-free text paper, manufactured in accordance with the proposed ANSI/NISO Z39.48-199X and ANSI Z39.48-1984

Contents

Preface

In 1982, a close relative was admitted to a teaching hospital 'somewhere in England'. On visiting him at 11 o'clock one morning, his untouched breakfast sat where it had been left, out of his reach, by the door. Unwashed, and humiliated at being in a wet bed, he was nearly in tears. He had been unable to ring for help because the nurses had placed his buzzer out of reach, because (he said) they had told him he was using it too much. On approaching one of the four staff chatting at the nurses' station to ask for extra pillows to enable us to sit him up to help his breathing, we were told 'You must be joking, they are like gold-dust round here'.

One word cropped up repeatedly in our subsequent letter of complaint regarding the care he received in hospital. This was 'Quality'. At the time, this concept was relatively unexplored territory for nursing in the UK. This was soon to change, with the introduction of Quality Assurance, Nursing Audit, Standard Setting and, most recently, Total Quality Management; all of which demanded time and effort from nurses in clinical practice.

Like many nurses, we initially met these new initiatives with scepticism and resistance. After all, we were much too busy looking after patients to devote any time to all this 'new fangled stuff'. But then, the staff on the ward 'somewhere in England' probably said that too.

This book describes our efforts to introduce Quality Improvement into clinical nursing, based on our practical experiences in using a variety of different approaches. The chapters follow the order in which we were introduced to these new ideas, as we suspect that, for many other clinically based nurses, their first exposure to 'Quality' is through involvement in setting standards.

Chapter 1 therefore outlines some different approaches to standard setting, and explains how these approaches were used by a multidisciplinary team in setting a standard for patient discharge.

Setting standards proved to be a productive and worthwhile exercise, but we soon realized that we had no way of knowing whether or not these actually had any impact on clinical practice. This could only be established by the use of some kind of audit. Chapter 2 therefore introduces nursing audit, and explains its application into practice through the use of case studies.

Audit identified whether or not our standards were being met, but it soon became apparent that many other areas were carrying out similar work, and some efforts were being duplicated. There was also a potential problem that staff would set clinically unsound standards, and these would not be identified, as there was no official system for approving the standards. We were also aware that a number of audit tools had become available commercially and could prove useful to us.

Chapter 3 therefore explains the use of Quality Assurance as a method for monitoring and co-ordinating not only nursing standards, but other Quality Assurance tools.

This worked well for a while, but we became aware that, in some areas, the same deficiencies identified through Quality Assurance cropped up repeatedly. Our problem was that we had approached Quality Assurance as an end in itself, rather than a means to an end. There was little point in auditing, (and creating a bureaucracy to manage this) if clinical practice did not improve as a result. It became apparent to us that there was a need to be able to plan and manage change if practice was to improve. At the same time that we realized this there was also a strong movement in the UK to adopt the method of care delivery referred to as 'Primary Nursing', as an attempt to improve the quality of patient care (Manthey, 1980). The process of managing the change to Primary Nursing was one of the most complex of our careers.

Chapter 4 therefore reviews the literature on the theories of change management and Chapter 5 then explains how we used these to help us to introduce Primary Nursing. The focus of these Chapters is intentionally practical, and is aimed at Clinical Nurses who have read the theories but (like ourselves at the time) are unsure how to integrate these into clinical practice.

As time progressed, in spite of us having implemented all these useful initiatives, with significant improvements in clinical practice as a result, there were still a large number of Quality problems that remained unresolved. Patient waiting lists were still too long, waiting times in clinics and Casualty often ran into hours, pillows were still 'like gold-dust'.

'The system' seemed to be designed with the sole intention of creating as much hassle as possible for the nurses attempting to deliver Quality care to the patients. It slowly dawned on us that further Quality Improvement could only be realized by extending our efforts beyond the nursing domain.

Chapter 6 therefore introduces an organizational approach to managing quality improvement referred to as Total Quality Management. The chapter begins with a precis of some of the common themes running through the differing approaches to Total Quality Management. This is followed by a series of short vignettes on some of the well-known authorities on this subject. Chapter 7 is devoted to outlining how one such approach was implemented in a hospital. Again, the focus of this case study is

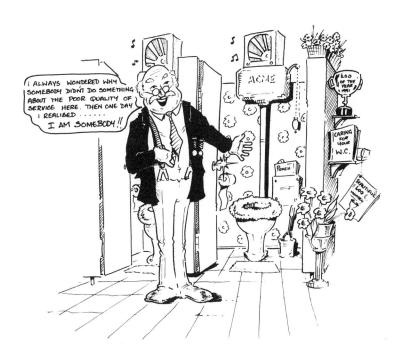

deliberately practical and descriptive. It is aimed at giving an insight into what the practical application of Total Quality Management in a hospital can involve. This was information that was extremely difficult to come by when we first became interested in this approach. There were a number of sources outlining what Total Quality Management is (referenced in Chapter 7) but a paucity of literature on how to implement the various concepts so they became part of the established organizational culture.

Like the nurses on the ward 'somewhere in England', it is all too easy to fall into the trap of accepting and delivering a poor quality of service. When faced with less than adequate resources, staff shortages and a plethora of other daily problems, it is easy to feel like a very small, insignificant cog in a very large, overwhelming wheel. After all, what difference can one individual make?

This was the first quantum leap we had to make when embarking on the process of Quality Improvement, as shown in the Illustration. When it comes to Quality Improvement, everyone has a role to play. In the words of the Chinese proverb. 'If you are not part of the solution, you are a part of the problem.'

REFERENCE

Manthey, M. (1980) _The Practice of Primary Nursing_. Blackwell Scientific, Boston.

Acknowledgements

The authors are indebted to Dr Keith Hurst, George English, John Parsley and Gerry Corrigan for their support and advice in compiling this manuscript; and to colleagues past and present who have enthusiastically contributed towards the numerous initiatives outlined in this book.

1

An introduction to setting standards

The link between Quality and some kind of 'standard' is not new. It crops up regularly in the media, with references being made to standards 'rising' or 'falling'. The word 'standards' was used in a similar context at our meetings, which were designed to address the issue of quality in nursing. When questioned further, many staff were unable to define these 'standards', or to put any quantifiable measure to them to prove that they were rising or falling; this was something that was just 'felt'.

We likened this approach to being told to go and jump over an invisible wall (Illustration 1.1). On enquiring how high the wall was, the answer was 'I'll tell you when you've jumped over it!' So it was with clinical practice. Often, we were given no clear guidelines on what was expected of us, and found out what the 'standard' was only when we failed to meet it.

Pressure area care was a good example of lack of a clear standard resulting in the use of a variety of different approaches. These included rubbing oil and spirit onto patients' heels and ankles, and whisking up a pavlova mix and placing it on patients' buttocks whilst applying oxygen. There was a consensus that there had to be a 'best' way of carrying out this important aspect of nursing care, but no one was sure what it was.

Defining standards provides a clear definition of an agreed level of performance for practitioners, and offers a measure against which current practice can be compared. There are two important areas of consideration when attempting to set standards. First, there is a need to select a framework that enables those setting standards to consider all the various components necessary for meeting that standard (Donabedian, 1969; Maxwell, 1984; Crosby, 1989). Second, consideration also needs

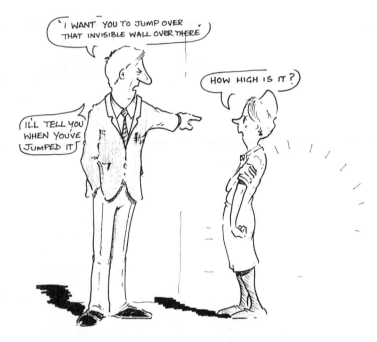

Illustration 1.1 The invisible wall.

to be given as to who should actually be setting the standards, and how this whole process is to be co-ordinated. These are explored below.

AN INTRODUCTION TO STANDARD-SETTING FRAMEWORKS

A number of different frameworks can be used to set standards. Of these, the Donabedian 'structure, process, outcome', has been most widely adopted by the nursing profession (Donabedian, 1969). This framework is outlined below. Three other frameworks are also explored in this Chapter; the Crosby Process model worksheet, Maxwell's six dimensions of quality; and criteria listing (Crosby, 1989; Maxwell, 1984). Each of these is used to formulate a multidisciplinary discharge standard to explore the practical application of each framework, and to examine the differences and similarities between them.

The Donabedian 'structure, process, outcome' framework

Donabedian first published his framework for setting standards in 1969. His approach has been adopted, over 20 years later, by the nursing profession, with further development of the framework and production of a comprehensive teaching package by the Royal College of Nursing Standards Of Care Project Team (1990). Much of the pioneering work in this field was done by Kitson (1988 a,b) Kendall (1988) and Howell and Marr (1988).

The next section introduces the terminology used and guidelines for using this approach. Its practical application is then discussed through using a case study of a multidisciplinary team's attempt at developing a standard for patient discharge planning.

Writing the standard statement

The first part of formulating a written standard involves defining the 'standard statement', which describes the objectives of the standard. An example of such a statement is 'The Charge Nurse will ensure all new staff on Nightingale ward receive instruction on safe lifting and handling techniques by the physiotherapist within 5 days of commencing employment.'

There are some important factors to consider when developing the standard statement (RCN, 1990):

- *The standard statement should have a clearly defined target group (or resource) at whom the standard is aimed.* This is important for two reasons. First, it identifies clearly, to individuals who are involved in meeting the standard, who or what the standard applies to. In the above example, this is 'All new staff on Nightingale ward'. In instances where the standard is not aimed at client or staff groups, but at resources, the target group should be similarly stated. For example 'All the wheelchairs in the outpatient department' or 'All the hospital budget statements'.

  Second, it identifies the sample group that needs to be audited to see whether the standard is being met. (The process of auditing standards is discussed in more detail in Chapter 2.)

- *The standard statement should state which individual, or group of individuals, is responsible for maintaining the standard.* This is important, as it places an onus of responsibility for meeting the standard with specific individuals, or groups (for example 'All trained staff'). In the above example, the responsibility for teaching the nurses rests with the physiotherapist. The responsibility for ensuring the nurse attends lies with the charge nurse. In the event of the standard not being met, it is the responsibility of these two individuals to take action to rectify the problem. If the action required falls outside their sphere of responsibility, then it is up to them to inform others of the deficiency who are able to help. In the above example, if the ward is short staffed, the Charge Nurse will need to report this to the manager and ask for relief to enable the nurse to attend the lecture.

  Failure to include spheres of responsibility in this way can cause problems in meeting the standard. In practice, we have found this can lead to situations where everyone assumes the responsibility to meet the standard will be carried by someone else.

- *The standard statement should be within the sphere of influence of those setting the standard.* If standard-setting is to improve clinical practice, it is essential that the components of the standard can be met by those writing them. For example, nurses may write a technically excellent standard for planning patient discharge. However, to implement all the criteria, they require at least 48 hours notice that the patient can go home (so that they can book appropriate community support, transport home, and complete relevant Health Education Programmes). Medical staff may be unaware of this, and normal practice may be to tell the patients on the ward round they can go home on that same day. The standard cannot therefore be met. A solution to this problem is to include other professionals whose co-operation is required in developing the standard.

- *The standard statement should be a clear statement of intent.* There is no place in standard statements for 'weasel words'. These are phrases that attempt to 'weasel out' of committing oneself to the standard. For example, 'The Charge Nurse will endeavour to ensure that most new staff on Nightingale ward receive instruction on safe lifting and handling techniques by the physiotherapist; preferably within 5 days of commencing employment'. Weasel words make it difficult to measure the standard (in the last example there is no mandatory requirement to attend a lifting lecture because of the use of 'preferably' and 'endeavour' and 'most'). They also absolve individuals of their responsibility for maintaining the standard, because they are not definitive.

Providing the standard meets the five criteria outlined below, it should be possible to compile a definitive statement.

Guidelines for formulating standard statements and criteria statements

Criteria statements provide the detailed information on how the standard statement is to be achieved. They are discussed in more detail on page 8.

Standard statements and criteria statements should be SMART, namely Specific, Measurable, Achievable, Relevant and Theoretically based:

- *Specific* The standard statement and criteria statements should be clear, understandable and unambiguous. When writing specific statements and criteria, it helps to consider the following questions:
  (i) *Why* is the standard being written? The most common reason for setting a standard is that staff have identified a problem. Focusing on the root cause of the problem can ensure that criteria are included in the standard to eliminate the problem. For example, the above standard may have been written as a result of an excessive number of lifting injuries sustained by nurses. Investigation found none of those injured had received instruction on lifting techniques. This can therefore be incorporated into the standard. Other reasons for writing standards include areas of interest, an area for improvement or a new idea or service that appears desirable.
  (ii) *What* is the standard statement or criteria statement referring to? This should be stated in specific terms. For example, 'Patients will be nursed with appropriate available equipment', is non-specific. It does not tell the

reader which patients the standard refers to, or what equipment is deemed appropriate. Conversely, 'All patients with a hemiplegia will be given a plateguard and wide-handled cutlery at mealtimes' is much more specific.

(iii) *Who* is involved? This should include the individual or group for whom the standard is written, and the individual or group who need to take action to meet the standard.

(iv) *When* should specific criteria be met? This falls into two categories. First, specific timings for actions that are stated in the standard. In the above example, all new nurses should attend the lifting lecture 'within 5 days'. Other examples include criteria that need to occur on a regular basis, such as 'daily' or 'twice weekly'. It is quite clear to those reading such criteria when, or how often, they are expected to comply with them. Second, the timing for implementation of the standard needs to be discussed. Those writing the standard should set a target date for its being met and should plan an audit shortly after this date to measure the impact of the new standard.

(v) *How* will the standard statement be met? This needs to consider the structure criteria, process criteria and outcome criteria necessary for meeting the standard statement.

(vi) *Where* does the overall standard apply to? This can range from one specific ward to a hospital or regional standard.

- *Measurable* Unless the standard statement and criteria statements are measurable, there is no way of knowing whether the standard is being met. If the standard statement is measurable, but the criteria statements are unmeasurable, it is impossible to establish the reasons for failure in the event of the standard statement not being met. For example, the standard statement may state 'Patients on Ward 2 will remain free from pressure sores'. This can be measured easily. The criteria statements may include 'The nurse will turn the patient when necessary'; or 'Appropriate pressure relieving aids will be used'. These are subjective and unmeasurable. Opinions may vary as to what constitutes 'appropriate' or 'when necessary'. Therefore, if patients on Ward 2 develop pressure sores, staff will not know why. Conversely, 'Patients identified at risk on a Pressure Score Rating Scale will be turned 2 hourly' is specific and measurable. Formulating specific criteria is the easiest way of ensuring they are measurable.

• *Achievable* Opinion differs as to where the benchmark for standards should lie. Some consider that 'minimum standards' should be written, i.e. establishing the lowest acceptable standards. Others believe that standards should reflect what happens in practice. A third approach to determining the standard involves defining an optimum level, which the practitioner strives to attain. Our own belief is that standards should be set to meet the requirements of the customer. These will include the mandatory requirements (as defined by the professionals) for acceptable practice. Professional input is needed to identify the technical aspects of care that the customer is unable to define. For example, a patient with abdominal pain will not be able to identify the technical requirements to ensure that they have a successful operation. However, the patient will have requirements relating to their environment and comfort, such as adequate postoperative analgesia and assistance with hygiene. This may mean challenging current practice and attempting to secure increased resources. Underpinning this approach is the concept of quality improvement and how one defines the term 'quality'. Using the example of pressure area care, we believe this needs to be done correctly 100% of the time. 'Minimum' implies something less than this. Similarly, there are dangers in documenting the standard currently adopted if this falls short of what is acceptable professional practice (for example rubbing oil and spirit into pressure areas). This is not to encourage the writing of unrealistic standards. There is little point in deciding that all patients will be nursed in a penthouse suite and cared for by six nurses every shift. However, this is easy to avoid if the point made above (regarding setting standards that are within the sphere of influence of those compiling them) is adhered to and if requirements are clearly identified.

• *Relevant* All the criteria statements in the standard should be relevant to meeting the standard statement. For the above example, the criteria statement 'The nurse will sign her contract on the first day of appointment' is irrelevant to meeting the standard of attending the lifting lecture within 5 days of starting the new job. In practice, we have found that irrelevant criteria often slip into standards if the standard statement is non-specific or ambiguous (Evans and Corrigan, 1990).

• *Theoretically sound* The standard statement and criteria statement should be theoretically sound. This covers several areas:
(i) Clinical criteria should be based on current research findings.
(ii) They should reflect the professional code of conduct, as defined by the professional bodies.
(iii) They should incorporate legal and statutory requirements.
(iv) They should be ethical.

The above guidelines are important for the standard statement and the criteria statements. The latter will now be explored in more detail.

Donabedian referred to three different types of criteria necessary to meet the standard: (i) structural criteria; (ii) process criteria; and (iii) outcome criteria. We have found the easiest way to understand these is to use the analogy of baking a cake. The standard statement might be 'An edible 10-inch chocolate sponge cake will be delivered to C ward before 6 p.m. every Friday'.

Structure criteria
These describe the resources in the system that are required to meet the standard, they include:

• Equipment (the oven, mixer, cooking utensils).
• Buildings (the kitchen).
• Staff (the cook).
• Agreed policies and procedures (the recipe, health and safety procedures).
• Ancillary services (the porter to deliver the cake).
• Materials (eggs, flour, etc.).

Process criteria
These describe the actions required by individuals in order to meet the standard, they include:

- Actions in implementing and monitoring the standard (for example, the cook reads the recipe, the cook weighs the ingredients; the cook mixes the ingredients).
- Assessment technique and procedure (for example, the cook assesses the oven temperature, the cook follows health and safety guidelines).
- Education, training and knowledge needed to meet the standard (for example, the cook has a City and Guild certificate; the cook shows subordinates how to bake the cake).
- Methods of giving information (for example, the ward sends a written request for the cake on Wednesday before 6 p.m.).
- Evaluation activities to be performed by those involved in meeting the standard (for example, the cook checks that the cake is cooked).

Outcome Criteria
These describe the desired effect of the standard in terms of behaviour, responses, level of knowledge and satisfaction (for example, 'An edible 10-inch chocolate cake will arrive on C ward every Friday before 6 p.m.' or 'The cook's subordinates will demonstrate their ability to bake a chocolate sponge cake').

Case study

This case study applies the 'structure, process, outcome' framework in setting a multidisciplinary standard for patient discharge from hospital.

A multidisciplinary team was convened to set a standard aimed at improving discharge planning within the hospital. The team consisted of all of those professionals who were involved in planning and co-ordinating discharge of patients from hospital.

The first task was to compile a standard statement that took account of the guidelines listed above. This proved difficult for two reasons. First, the term 'discharge' proved ambiguous. We were unsure whether this included patients discharged to other hospitals and of where the 'discharge' started or finished (for example, was it when the patient left the hospital gates, when they arrived home safely or when they returned for their first outpatient appointment?).

Second, we found it hard to set a standard that we could guarantee we could achieve. Impressive statements such as 'All patients will have their socioeconomic and health needs met on discharge from hospital.' had to be discarded when we realized that they were outside our sphere of influence. If the patients wanted to go home to unsuitable circumstances, and to disregard all our well-intended health education, this was their privilege. Our role (it was decided) was to ensure patients were offered the components of a planned discharge to enable them to make an informed choice. Providing we did this, the choice was then with the patient. A statement that met the SMART criteria as closely as possible is shown on the completed standard in Table 1.1. The term 'planned' referred to the criteria stated in the standard, and to the multidisciplinary discharge procedure.

The structural components were then determined. This process involved all the professionals who had a role to play in planning patient discharge. This resulted immediately in one problem – the social worker was leaving, and no immediate replacement was available.

The team debated other structural components, such as buildings and equipment. It was decided not to include all the wards and departments, telephones, typewriters, etc. as these were too numerous to mention. Also, it was felt at the time that the problems had arisen because of lack of an established system for planning patient discharges, rather than shortage of materials or equipment. The decision was taken to include specific essential items in the multidisciplinary discharge procedure, rather than in the standard.

During the discussions it became apparent that no clear procedure incorporated all the disciplines relating to patient discharge. This was causing problems, as some aspects of patient discharge had never been assigned to a specific discipline. For example, everyone agreed that it was necessary to liaise with local authority rehabilitation officers for provision of disability equipment, house adaptations and other support services, but it had never been established who should do this. The team also became aware that even where there was an established procedure (such as in nursing), many staff were unaware of it, and some parts of the procedure required updating.

There was clearly a need for a multidisciplinary discharge procedure to resolve these issues. Initially we were confused between what constituted a standard and what constituted a

Table 1.1 Discharge standard using the Donabedian framework

Standard Statement: All patients in 'X' hospital will have their discharge from hospital planned by the multidisciplinary team

Structure	Process	Outcome
• A multidisciplinary team including: consultant, senior house officer, RGN, community liaison sister, occupational therapist, physiotherapist, speech therapist, dietitian, social worker • Staff pharmacist • Medical secretary • Medical records clerk • Ambulance service • A multidisciplinary discharge procedure	• The multidisciplinary team will assess the patient's social, medical and physical needs prior to discharge • Members of the multidisciplinary team will follow the discharge procedure and maintain the discharge standard • Members of the multidisciplinary team will offer the patient information and advice outlined in the discharge procedure • Members of the multidisciplinary team will check the patient's understanding of information and advice • The members of the multidisciplinary team will document a written plan of discharge for the patient • The multidisciplinary team will audit the standard every 6 months	• All discharges will be planned • Comunication within the multidisciplinary team is improved • The patient's social, medical and physical needs are met on discharge • Discharges are audited • The score on the audit tool will improve

procedure; an extremely common mistake to make when neither of these two documents exist. Broadly speaking, a procedure describes actions that need to be performed by an individual to complete a given task. A standard is a professionally agreed level of performance aimed at a particular population that meets the five components of the SMART guidelines. Hence the discharge procedure was required to inform individuals within each discipline of the actions they were required to undertake when discharging a patient. For example 'The nurse will ensure the patient's valuables are returned to him or her on discharge'. The discharge standard was required to define an agreed level of service that patients discharged from hospital could expect to receive.

In the absence of a procedure it is common to find procedural statements being incorporated into the standard. This was our first big mistake; with the initial standard being 12 pages long. This was resolved by starting again, and writing a separate multidisciplinary discharge procedure, which was then mentioned under the 'structure' column as a document that was essential for meeting the standard, so it was not necessary to repeat these criteria in the standard itself.

The process criteria were then compiled. These had to be done to meet the standard, and are shown in Table 1.1. They proved relatively straightforward. A key consideration here was the need for both documents to be 'active' and not left to sit on a shelf and gather dust. This was resolved by including a representative from all areas as a link person, to explain the new standard and procedure to all staff. At a later date it was realized the impact of these could only be effectively monitored through the use of an audit tool. This was also included under the process element of the standard.

The outcome criteria were then agreed, as shown in Table 1.1. These were more difficult to formulate using the SMART criteria, as many of the original criteria suggested were subjective, impossible to measure or outside the sphere of influence of the team. The final five criteria were agreed, with the agreement on the meaning of these as follows:

- Outcome 1 'All discharges will be planned' referred to all the criteria within the discharge standard and discharge procedure being met.

- Outcome 2 'Communication within the multidisciplinary team is improved' seemed a reasonable expectation in the light of the work that had been done by the group. This could be measured by a questionnaire to ascertain the views of staff as to whether the discharge standard and procedure had led to specific improvements in communications between disciplines. It was also measured in the audit tool, which included criteria such as the amount of notice nurses were given by Medical staff that the patient was to be discharged, and whether social workers received referrals.
- Outcome 3 'The patient's social, medical and physical needs were met in discharge'. This was rejected as the standard statement as it was felt to be outside the sphere of influence of the team in the event of a patient refusing these services. However, it was felt to be a reasonable expected outcome. The important factor was that all of these areas had been assessed, with the patient being offered the appropriate treatment or service. It was these factors that were measured in the audit tool.
- Outcomes 4 and 5 referred to the use of the audit tool, and the expectation that the score should improve with the implementation of the standard.

General comments on the practical application of this model

The Donabedian framework has several advantages when setting a standard. The first involves the ownership of the standard by those setting it, and the improved communications that arose from this exercise. We found the framework a useful method for considering the different components required to meet the standard. Formulating the standard statement first helped in establishing relevant criteria required to meet the standard.

There were some difficulties within the context of setting this particular standard. First, due to the more abstract nature of the standard, it was difficult to identify structural components. There is a difference of opinion as to how this component is addressed by those using the standard. Some advocate the use of this column to identify factors such as staff knowledge and information (RCN 1990). Others refer to Donabedian's initial intention that structural factors should be those that do not change (such as buildings and equipment) and argue that knowledge and staffing levels can change from structure or process depending on one's position within the organization (Goldstone, 1991). This raises the problem of deciding which criteria belong in which column. Our final conclusion was that, providing relevant criteria were identified (in terms of practical application of the standard), it made no difference whether criteria were listed in the structure, process or outcome column.

The second difficulty lay in the implied relationship that the three columns have with each other. Initially we made the mistake of trying to use the standard form layout shown in Table 1.1 as a flow sheet, where structural, process and outcome components were all linked across the page. We then identified the problem (as in the example of the non-compliant patient) that the structure and process criteria may all be met, but the outcome is not. This proved particularly problematic in our initial attempts at auditing outcome measures and was resolved by incorporating measures of structure, process and outcome in the audit tool, which proved a far more effective indicator as to how the standard was working. The converse of this scenario can also present similar problems. For example, patients may achieve remarkable outcomes that mask the fact that the structural and process components are inadequate. Studies attempting to demonstrate a relationship between these three components have identified a poor, or non-existent, relationship between outcome measures and structural and process inputs (Overton and Stinson, 1977).

From an organizational perspective, widespread generation of a large number of standards proved logistically difficult to administrate. In the absence of a clearly defined mechanism for approving and maintaining the standards, their effectiveness can be impeded. At one extreme is the danger of poor standards being formulated and accepted locally, in the absence of organizational and professional guidance and control. At the other extreme, standards that reflect current research and good practice may be set, but cannot be implemented because of a lack of management commitment necessary to release funding and resources.

Absence of central co-ordination also led to a significant amount of duplication, with common interest areas such as Care Planning, Wound Care and Pressure Sore Prevention producing numerous variations of the same theme. This in turn creates the danger of conflicting standards arising within one unit.

The Crosby process model worksheet

The process model worksheet is one of the tools used in the Crosby approach to total quality management (TQM), which is explained through the use of a case study in Chapter 7. It is included in this chapter as another framework that can be used to set standards. The Crosby approach also advocates the use of 'flow-charting', which can be used to ascertain standards criteria. This is outlined briefly on page 19, as it is our experience that it can be used with any of the standard setting approaches mentioned in this chapter, and may prove useful to those attempting to develop an eclectic approach to standard setting.

Crosby uses slightly different terminology, referring to 'requirements' instead of 'standards'. His process model worksheet is designed to establish the requirements (or standards) for a given 'process'. Central to this approach is the underlying concept that 'All work is a process: a series of actions that produce a result' (Crosby, 1989). This means that, for all work processes, there will be inputs and outcomes, and customers and suppliers; as shown in the process model worksheet in Figure 1.1. For example, in the process 'discharging a patient', the 'outcome' will be the patient being discharged. The inputs will be all the materials, information, facilities, equipment, training, knowledge, procedures and performance standards that are needed to achieve the desired result.

The notion of the 'customer and supplier' is one that is used in many approaches to total quality management. Processes have four types of 'customer': (i) internal; (ii) external; (iii) immediate; and (iv) ultimate. A 'customer' is a recipient of a service or product at a given stage of the process.

'Internal' customers are all the individuals who are internal to the organization. In the process of discharging a patient, these would include the nurses and doctors.

'External' customers are those individuals external to the organization who receive goods or services as part of the

1 PROCESS NAME

Discharge of patients from hospital

2 SCOPE

Initial activity:
Consultant gives notice of discharge

Final activity:
Patient established in planned location

3

OUTCOMES	CUSTOMER	REQUIREMENT
Patient disharged from hospital	Patient	Planned by MDT • with all materials and equipment • on time • to correct location
3A	3B	3C

4

	INPUTS	SUPPLIERS	REQUIREMENTS
4a	*Materials* Drugs Valuables Patient transfer form	Pharmacy General office Nursing	Correct. 2 h notice Returned complete, on time Accurate/complete/on time
4b	*Information* Notice of discharge Patient's social status Patient's physical status Patient's medical status	Doctor Patient/Soc.work Patient/Nurse Doctor	12 h notice } Accurate On time Documented
4c	*Patient*	Consultant	Informed of discharge Involved in plan

Process controls

5 FACILITIES & EQUIPMENT

FACILITIES & EQUIPMENT	WHO PROVIDES	REQUIREMENTS
Ambulance	Ambulance service	48 h notice Arrives on time
Storage of drugs	Management	Conforms to drug storage procedure
Internal transport	Porters	1 h notice Arrives on time 48 h of notice of withdrawal
Secure place for money	General office	Returned on time

6 TRAINING & KNOWLEDGE

TRAINING & KNOWLEDGE	WHO PROVIDES	REQUIREMENTS
Discharge procedure	MDT/management	All staff aware of procedure All staff follow procedure
Induction for new staff re. discharge procedure	Departmental head	Within 2 days of appointment
Discharge audit tool	MDT	Used every 6 months

7 PROCEDURES

PROCEDURES	WHO DEFINES	REQUIREMENTS
MDT Discharge procedure	MDT (approved by management)	Includes crown guidelines • current • validated • agreed • available

8 PERFORMANCE STANDARDS

PERFORMANCE STANDARDS	WHO DEFINES	REQUIREMENTS
Quality	Professionals, management	Right first time
Cost	Professionals, management	Within budget
Schedule	Professionals management	On time

*MDT, multidisciplinary team.

Figure 1.1 Discharge process using the Process model worksheet.

process. In the process of discharging a patient, these would include the General Practitioner, who receives the discharge summary of the care of their patient from the hospital doctor, and the patient.

The 'ultimate' customer is the individual who is the ultimate recipient of the service or product produced by the process. In the process of discharging a patient, the ultimate customer is the patient.

The 'immediate' customer refers to the recipient of the product or service during an intermediate stage of the process. In the process of discharging a patient, the Pharmacy would be a customer of the prescription chart stating the discharge medication of the patient.

All processes also have 'suppliers'. 'Supplier' refers to the individual or department that delivers essential goods or services necessary for the process. For example, the pharmacy department is a supplier of the drugs necessary for the patient on discharge. It can be appreciated that, within a given process, one can be both a customer and supplier. Hence the Pharmacist is a customer when receiving the completed drug chart specifying the discharge medication and a supplier when dispensing the medication.

When examining a process using this approach it is necessary to identify all the customers and suppliers within the process, because all these individuals need to agree the requirements necessary for making the process work (or, to use previous terminology, for meeting the standard). For example, the Pharmacist requires a certain amount of notice to enable the Pharmacy Department to prepare the drugs for the patient's discharge. However, when examining this process, it became apparent that, in a significant proportion of cases, the prescription was written at the last minute, with the nurse having to go to Pharmacy to collect the drugs. The amount of notice required by the Pharmacy to enable them to prepare the drugs had never been defined and, during this process, the Pharmacy was able to negotiate an acceptable amount of notice with the medical staff. The important factor in establishing requirements in this way is that they should be agreed between the customer and supplier. In cases where one area 'imposed' a new set of requirements without agreeing them with the supplier, they were (understandably) often never met. The benefit of establishing requirements in the process of discharging patients was that it gave all the individuals involved in the process an insight into the needs of their colleagues, which ultimately improved the process.

Establishing clear requirements is a useful precursor for auditing the process, as these are easily transferred into audit criteria. For example, if it is agreed that the Pharmacy requires 2 hours notice for discharge prescriptions, it can easily measure the number of times this requirement (or standard) is not met.

Flow-charting

Flow-charting can be useful to identify components that need to be included in the standard framework. Flow charts are also useful when examining work processes, as they enable the most likely source of potential problems in the process to be identified. Figure 1.2 shows an example of a flow chart completed by the multidisciplinary team dealing with one part of the discharge process – sending discharge letters to the patient's General Practitioner (GP) on discharge. The initial agreed requirement (agreed between the medical staff and medical records) was that these should reach the GP within 21 days of the patient being discharged. (A discharge summary was always sent on the day of discharge; the discharge letter was a more detailed account of the patient's progress in hospital.) Audit had identified that this requirement was not being met.

The flow chart shows the normal chain of events in the process of writing patient discharge letters. It identifies those involved in the process, the materials and equipment needed. Each stage offers potential clues as to where the errors in the system may be occurring. For example, in stage 2, if the notes are not available on the ward, the Doctor will be unable to complete the process. Further understanding of the process can be gained by involving those identified by the flow chart as part of the process in completing a process model work-sheet.

The flow chart also offers a useful framework for different disciplines to examine a process that crosses both professional or departmental interfaces, where each area only sees a small part of the overall process. There is typically little insight by many staff into the requirements of these other areas.

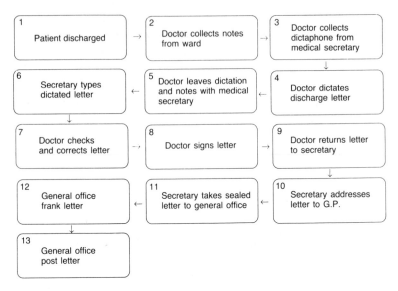

Figure 1.2 Flowchart showing process of compiling discharge letters to General Practitioners.

Completing the process model worksheet

For ease of explanation, the process model worksheet shown in Figure 1.1 is numbered in the order in which it is completed. Each of these steps is explained below:

1. *Process name*. This simply requires the name of the process under examination to be completed; in this case 'Discharge of patients from hospital'.

2. *Scope*. This refers to the scope of the process being examined. The simplest way to determine the scope is to refer back to the flow chart for the process. For example, in Figure 1.2, it may be the whole process that needs exploring, in which case the contents from the first box 'Patient discharged' are entered under 'Initial activity' and the last box 'General office post letter' under 'Final activity'. Conversely, one may wish to scrutinize a particular part of a complex process, and narrow the scope. For example, in Figure 1.2 one could have the initial activity as 'Doctor leaves dictation and notes with medical secretary', as shown in box 5, and the final activity as 'Doctor checks and corrects letter', as shown in box 7.

We think of determining the scope as similar to using a lens on a camera. One can either 'zoom in' and examine a certain part in more detail, or take a wide-angled look at the overall process. In our experience, we often tended to make the scope too large, which complicated the worksheet unnecessarily.

It was helpful to determine the scope for the process of discharging patients because, as mentioned earlier, many of us were unsure as to where the process started and finished. Initially, this led to us attempting to incorporate every conceivable criterion into the standard. The team finally decided that the initial activity was the Consultant giving notice that the patient was fit for discharge and that the final activity was that the patient was established in the planned location. The latter phrase was used to incorporate patients transferred to other hospitals or nursing homes.

3. *Outcomes.* It is necessary to consider the outcomes of the process prior to any inputs. Unless the outcomes of the process are clearly defined, it is difficult to establish what inputs are required. If you don't know what you want, you won't know what you need to get it!

In this example, the outcome of the process is the patient discharged, as shown in Figure 1.1 (3a).

Figure 1.1 (3b) asks who the customers of the outcome are. In this instance, it was limited to the patient, but there may be more than one customer for a given process. For example, another output that could be included from this process is the discharge letter; the customer in this instance would be the GP. Different customers will often have different requirements from the same process, as shown in Figure 1.1 (3c). The requirements of the patient are that:

(i) The discharge is planned by the multidisciplinary team with consideration of social, medical and physical needs.
(ii) The patient is discharged to the correct location.
(iii) The patient is given all necessary materials and equipment in preparation for discharge.
(iv) The patient is discharged on time.

If the letter to the GP had been included in this section the requirements would differ. They would be:

(i) The letter should arrive within 21 days.
(ii) The letter should be accurate.

(iii) The letter should be complete.
4. *Inputs.* This stage defines the material and information inputs required for the process. The model has been adapted for the health service to include a third box for the patient. This was because, for many of our processes, the patient is the 'input', and including them as a 'material' was regarded as inappropriate.

Material inputs (Figure 1.1 (4a)) are the inputs that are required by the process, and are altered or consumed in some way by the process. Returning to the earlier cake-baking analogy; the material inputs would be the eggs, sugar, flour, etc.

In this example, the material inputs are the drugs required on discharge, the money and valuables belonging to the patient that may be in safe keeping ('altered' by the process, as cash is returned as a cheque!) and the patient transfer form, which is altered by being written on.

The suppliers of the material inputs are indicated. This proved a useful method of agreeing clear areas of responsibility for supplying certain inputs essential to the process that had not previously been established. For example, the General Office agreed to return all money and valuables to the patient prior to discharge, but required 48 hours notice from nursing staff if a large cheque needed to be arranged.

The requirements for each of the material inputs are then agreed, as shown in the final box in Figure 1.1 (4a).

Information inputs (Figure 1.1 (4b)) is the information required to operate the process. In this instance, this relies on the Consultant informing the multidisciplinary team of the intention to discharge the patient; and information on the patient's social, physical and medical needs on discharge. The individuals responsible for supplying this information are shown in the following boxes. The requirements for each of these information inputs is shown in the final boxes.

The 'patient' input to the process (Figure 1.1 (4c)) identifies the supplier as the Consultant, because once he or she gives notice of discharge the process begins. The patient's requirements of this information are shown in the final box.
5. *Facilities and equipment.* This box identifies all the facilities and equipment necessary for the discharge process. These are things that need to be present but, unlike the material inputs,

are not altered or changed by the process. In the analogy of baking the cake, equipment would include the cake tin, the oven and the utensils, because these are 'left' at the end of the process. The facilities would include the portering service, to deliver the cake, and the Supplies Department to deliver the ingredients.

The facilities and equipment, as identified by the multi-disciplinary team for the discharge process are shown in box 5, along with the suppliers of these. Again, agreeing the requirements of these between different disciplines was an important part of improving the process.

6. *Training and knowledge.* It is at this stage that the staff required for the process are identified, along with any training or knowledge necessary for the process. This was a useful step, as it forced the team to consider how all staff would be informed of the new multidisciplinary discharge procedure. This was important if it was not to be filed away to gather dust with all the other procedures.

7. *Procedures.* This box identifies any procedure necessary for the process. These may be already established or, as in the case of the multidisciplinary standard, require developing. It was an interesting observation that, in many of the processes we examined using this model, there were few defined procedures for many work processes. Many were carried out 'because they'd always been done like that', or were carried out differently (as with pressure area care), depending on who was involved in the process.

8. *Performance standards.* This box determines the performance standard for quality, cost and schedule. Ideally, these should be defined by senior management and professionals. In terms of the performance standard for the quality of this process, the requirements identified should all be done 'right the first time'. The process should be carried out within the allocated budget, and the schedule for all the requirements identified is defined as all of them occurring 'on time'.

General comments on the practical application of this model

This framework also proved a useful method for identifying the different components necessary to meet the requirements in the process of discharging a patient. It concentrated the minds of the team on establishing requirements (or standards) for each of the components. This was useful both for improving the process, and for ensuring that requirements were measurable. The use of the 'scope' was found to be advantageous, as it forced us to focus on the specific part of the process that was causing us difficulty.

The framework itself is more comprehensively laid out than that of the Donabedian model. Some staff preferred the more explicit headings, whereas others felt it was too complicated and difficult to understand. Training in use of the model was an important factor in its ease of use, and this is referred to in more detail in the general conclusions.

Similar difficulties were identified to those highlighted with the Donabedian model on the implied relationship between structure, process and outcome.

Maxwell's dimensions of quality

Maxwell first published his 'dimensions of quality' in 1984. He identified six components that contribute towards quality standards:

- Access to service.
- Relevance to need.
- Effectiveness.
- Equity.
- Social acceptability.
- Efficiency and economy.

This framework can also be used in setting standards for patient discharge, as illustrated below.

Discharge standard using Maxwell's dimensions

- Access to service
    (i) All patients will have access to a fully planned discharge service, as defined in the multidisciplinary discharge procedure.
    (ii) Patients requiring transport on discharge, or for follow-up appointments, will have this arranged by nursing staff, and will be informed of arrival and departure times.

(iii) Patients requiring community services will have these arranged prior to discharge.

- Relevance to need
  (i) All members of the multidisciplinary team will assess the patient's social, medical and physical needs on discharge.
  (ii) The multidisciplinary team will discuss with the patient their perceived needs on discharge.
  (iii) Patients will be offered the components of a planned discharge to meet their individual needs.
- Effectiveness of the service
  (i) The multidisciplinary team will audit the discharge procedure every 6 months to ensure component criteria are met.
  (ii) The multidisciplinary team will audit circumstances relating to re-admission of patients to hospital within 1 week of discharge.
  (iii) A postdischarge survey will be undertaken to establish patient satisfaction with their discharge plan.
- Equity
  (i) All patients, regardless of sex, creed or colour, will be offed a planned discharge that takes account of their individual needs and the organization's ability to meet these needs. This may necessitate prioritization for the most needy.
  (ii) Non-English speaking patients requiring an interpreter will be supplied with one.
- Acceptability of service
  (i) The nurse will obtain feedback from the patient and relatives to ascertain the suitability of the discharge plan in meeting the individual needs of the patient.
- Efficiency and economy
  (i) A cost–benefit analysis will be completed to establish the impact of early discharge from hospital, and identify any necessary increase in community resources.
  (ii) A 'price of non-conformance' will be measured for this process, and actions taken to improve this cost.

General comments on the practical application of this model

Maxwell's dimensions offer an interesting alternative to the other two approaches outlined above. In the example of discharging a patient, it raised two areas previously unconsidered by the team; 'equity' and 'relevance to need.' One of the overriding problems identified by team members based in the community was their inability to meet the increasing demands placed upon them by patients being discharged earlier from hospital. This led ultimately to the prioritization of patients' demands.

'Relevance to need' was another new dimension. There was a danger that our well-intentioned attempts to offer everyone all the elements of a planned discharge would drastically increase the workload. However, many patients did not want a variety of professionals probing their social and economic circumstances, and many were quite content to go home and be left to their own devices. The role of the team was to ensure that those who required this service, received it.

This model could be particularly useful on a macro scale; such as when planning a new hospital or department. Its use is more limited on a smaller scale (for example, baking a cake, or as a standard for maintaining wheelchairs).

Disadvantages found in using this approach were that many of the dimensions tended to overlap, and similar criteria appeared in different dimensions. Developing audit tools on many of the criteria was markedly more difficult than for the other two approaches. Evaluating 'fairness' and 'acceptability' tended to be very subjective.

Criteria listing

This final method for writing standards is mentioned here because we are aware that, in spite of relatively little being published on this approach, many areas are using criteria listing as a way of defining standards. The quality assurance tools mentioned in Chapter 3 all consist of lists of standard criteria for assessment. Hence the standards are implicit within the clinical or organizational audit.

The guidelines for compiling standard criteria in the Donabedian model (namely they should be specific, measurable, achievable, relevant and theoretically based) also apply to this method. Using the discharge standard as an example, the following criteria list was compiled:

- All members of the multidisciplinary team will follow the discharge procedure.
- Members of the multidisciplinary team will assess the patient's social, medical, and physical needs prior to discharge.
- Members of the multidisciplinary team will offer the patient information and advice as outlined in the discharge procedure.
- Members of the multidisciplinary team will formulate a written discharge plan, based on the patient's individual needs, prior to discharge.
- The members of the multidisciplinary team will audit the discharge standard (using the audit tool), at 6-monthly intervals.

The main advantage of this approach is that it is easy to use, and easy to understand. This can be a benefit to staff, who find it time-consuming trying to fit criteria into the three frameworks outlined above. It is also relatively easy to audit such criteria.

The main problem with this approach is that it is only a superficial examination of a number of criteria that may, or may not, be important in meeting certain standards. The relationship with other criteria is never explored. In the event of criteria not being met, no insight is given as to why this may be the case. Conversely, the use of the Donabedian or Process Model Worksheet offers greater potential to identify all the elements necessary to meet the standard or requirements.

GENERAL CONCLUSIONS

In drawing general conclusions concerning the usefulness of these four approaches in clinical practice, it is necessary to consider four questions:

- How is the standard-setting process implemented?
- Who is setting the standards?
- What are the standard frameworks to be used for?
- Why are the standards being set?

The first two questions address issues relevant to all four standard-setting approaches. The second two questions address the appropriateness of the use of specific standard setting frameworks.

Implementing the standard-setting process (the how and the who)

Three approaches can be used to implement the standard-setting process: (i) top down; (ii) bottom up; or (iii) a combination of the two.

'Top down' refers to the situation where senior management directs the standard-setting initiative. This can take two forms, either senior management sets the standards, and then circulates these for implementation; or they instruct their subordinates to set standards. The advantage of this approach is that it requires management to act in the event of standards not being met as a result of certain components (such as staff or equipment) not being available; as their involvement in the standard's formulation requires a degree of commitment to ensure the standard is met. The disadvantage of this approach is that it is our experience that staff resent this power-coercive approach. This means standards written by management are never 'owned' by staff, and are doomed to gather dust in filing cabinets. Staff who are instructed to write either a specific standard or who are given a number of standards to produce are unlikely to develop much enthusiasm for the process.

'Bottom up' refers to the situation where staff involved in clinical practice set their own standards. The advantage of this approach is that staff are committed to the resultant standard, and motivated in ensuring it is met. The disadvantage is that lack of support from management concerning the standard may mean that the staff do not have the necessary resources to implement the standard. Lack of direction could result in the setting of standards based on local practice, rather than validated by research.

The best approach for ensuring the development and use of standards that improve clinical practice is a combination of the two; advocated by Quality Assurance frameworks, (RCN, 1990), by the Total Quality Management approach and by change management theories. Staff therefore set standards that are owned by them, but they are supported in this process by management, who offer appropriate education and resources as well as monitoring and approving the standards set. The resultant standard is therefore owned by both staff and management.

In our experience, it is essential that staff are educated in the various approaches to setting standards. There are a number of instances of which we are aware where staff have been expected to write standards with no guidance at all. Without education, the resultant standards are usually difficult to understand, impossible to measure and forgotten by staff as soon as they have fulfilled their obligation in writing them.

Choosing an approach (the what)

In choosing an approach for setting standards, it is important to consider what the selected framework is to be used for. It can be seen from using the discharge standard as a case study that different frameworks can identify a number of different criteria, although all relate to the same process. Typically, in a 'top down' approach, staff are instructed to use a specific framework. This creates two problems. First, staff may become blinkered in the one approach, and fail to consider some of the equally relevant components of others. Second, it is our experience that some frameworks may be more appropriate in some situations than others.

For example, the Donabedian framework is useful for standards that have clearly defined structural, process and outcome criteria, like the process model worksheet. However, criteria listing may be more appropriate for relatively simple standards. For example, a standard for changing an oxygen cylinder can be expanded painfully into 'structure' (the porter, the nurse, the cylinder, the checking book, etc.) 'process' (the nurse informs the porter, the porter changes the cylinder, etc.) and 'outcome', when all that was needed is a verbal agreement between the staff concerned that they will observe the cylinder whilst in use and change it when empty. Conversely, the difficulty with many of the criteria lists in the Quality Assurance tools is that they only inform staff what is going wrong; not why. If a more detailed examination of the components is required, one of the other three frameworks would be a more appropriate choice.

The process model worksheet is useful for analysing work processes that are causing problems, through the use of identifying and agreeing requirements. We found that, for many work processes, the requirements were absent or poorly defined. This commonly led to a breakdown in the process due to lack of understanding by individuals of what was expected of them (Illustration 1.2). Maxwell (1984) adds some new dimensions that are particularly useful when examining organizational standards, such as for a new unit or service.

The other commonly made mistake is to attempt to write a standard when what is really required is a procedure, a policy or a protocol.

In examining the benefits of one standard-setting framework over another, comparisons can be drawn with the chequered history of the introduction of nursing models. There is a variety to choose from. Some are better validated than others; some lend themselves more easily to certain settings than others and some are more easily understood than others. Considering these factors, it would seem sensible to develop an eclectic approach to standard-setting, based on the individual standard being compiled. It would seem unreasonable to advocate one approach over and above all the others at this early stage of developing the art and science of setting standards.

Why set standards at all?

Some of the reasons for setting standards are outlined earlier in this chapter. It is important to establish at a local level the reason for setting standards. In our experience, if this is done to score 'brownie points' or to attempt to force reluctant individuals to change entrenched practice, the whole exercise is likely to fail.

Conversely, getting a group of staff together with a common interest, and in the presence of a supportive management, and educating them in the use of a framework can create a climate where any of the above tools offer a powerful vehicle for improving quality.

The main reason for setting standards should be to improve the quality of service. Standards are intended to be a dynamic tool to achieve this end. As such, it is not so much the framework used but the change that occurs in the perception and attitudes of those involved in writing the standard that will cause improvement to occur.

We found standard-setting on its own was insufficient for these changes in perception and attitudes to occur. Objective measurement of how performance rated in comparison to the

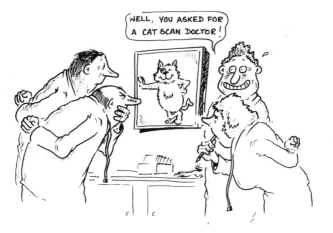

Illustration 1.2 What the doctor ordered.

agreed standard was essential in gaining recognition of the need to improve. This can only be achieved through auditing the standard that has been set, and taking action to rectify the deficiencies identified.

In conclusion, the setting of standards in itself is not enough; it is the first step on a long journey. One needs to develop audit tools to measure the standard to enable the cycle of Quality Improvement to begin. The use of audit, and an explanation of how it can be introduced into clinical practice, can be found in Chapter 2.

REFERENCES

Crosby, P. (1989) *Quality Education System for the Individual.* The Creative Factory, Crosby Quality College, London.

Donabedian, A. (1969) Evaluating the quality of medical care. *Millbank Memorial Fund Quarterly*, **4**, 166–203.

Evans, K. and Corrigan, P. (1990) Standard setting, an introduction to differing approaches. *Nursing Standard*, **May 22nd.**

Goldstone, L. (1991) A very peQALIar practice. *Nursing Times*, **87** (20).

Howell, J. and Marr, H. (1988) Visible improvements. *Nursing Times*, **84** (25), 33–4.

Kendall, H. (1988) The West Berkshire approach. *Nursing Times*, **84** (27) 33–4.

Kitson, A. (1988a) Raising the standards. *Nursing Times*, **84**(25), 29–32.

Kitson, A. (1988b) Caring standards. *Nursing Standard*, **November 5th.**

Kitson, A. (1989) *A Framework for Quality.* Scutari, London.

Maxwell, R.J. (1984) Quality assessment in health. *British Medical Journal*, **288** (5), 1470–2.

Overton, P. and Stinson, S. (1977) *Journal of Advanced Nursing*. **2**, 137–46.

Royal College of Nursing Standards of Care Project Team (1990) *Quality Patient Care, The Dynamic Standard Setting System*. Scutari, London.

2

Audit

INTRODUCTION

Chapter 1 established that the setting of standards is the first step in a long journey on the road of quality improvement. From a personal perspective, the first navigational difficulties along the way occurred as the ink was drying on our newly formulated standard sheets.

Setting standards in isolation seemed of little value if we had no means of knowing whether we were achieving them. There was a danger of viewing standard-setting as an end in itself, rather than a means to an end. If we were to arrive at our destination of quality improvement in clinical practice, it was important that we developed a mechanism that enabled us both to monitor standards and to take action to improve these standards where deficiencies were discovered.

It was this realization that led to our first exposure of 'audit'. This was a term being used increasingly at conferences and in the nursing journals to describe a whole host of activities. Common to this range of activities was an attempt to measure some aspect of nursing practice. There the similarities ended. Our literature search indicated a number of different approaches, which fell loosely into the following categories:

- Audit can take place by using off the shelf tools such as Monitor (Goldstone et al., 1983, 1984) Phaneufs (1976) or Qualpacs (Wandelt and Ager, 1984). It can be used on a systematic basis by the yearly auditing of a ward or department, or simply in response to an identified problem.
- The audit tools mentioned above aim to measure the quality of care, or are indicators of quality, either retrospectively or concurrently. Each is discussed in more detail later.

- Other methods of 'auditing' include criteria-based audits, such as 'infection control' (Horner, 1991) and those related to self-medication (Corrigan, 1991; Raycroft, 1991). These audits arose as a result of the identification of a problem requiring data collection, further assessment of the problem, implementation of a change strategy, evaluation and follow-up of the solution.
- Auditing can also include the identification of components necessary to deliver a high quality of nursing care, such as the framework offered by Donabedian (1976), which defines structure, process and outcome criteria.
- Audit is important when assessing the impact of a nursing innovation, such as the effect of a Nursing Development Unit, as there are limited funds available and the pressure to demonstrate results from various projects has increased. A framework indictating the ways in which effective auditing may be achieved is outlined below.

TYPES OF AUDIT USED BY NURSES

Research studies

At the academic end of the scale are the full-blown, properly conducted research projects. The feasibility of many grass-roots staff receiving both the funding and time to complete such projects in their own areas should never be excluded but, in reality, it is not an option available to many clinical nurses.

It is essential that research studies are not left to gather dust on a library shelf; practitioners should be active in seeking out relevant research papers and should incorporate relevant findings into their daily activities as a method of improving the quality of patient care. The communication links between researchers and practitioners desperately need improving.

It is possible for some ward-based staff to carry out small-scale research studies and still produce a relevant, valid and replicable study. These are to be encouraged, and there is help available for interested staff in the form of a wide range of excellent texts (Polit and Hungler, 1990), a growing number of short courses on research techniques and locally organized research interest groups.

Off the shelf audit tools

In recent years, a number of audit tools have become commercially available for use by nurses. These fall broadly into two categories: (i) those that attempt to measure quantitative aspects of nursing, focusing on workload dependence systems; and (ii) those that attempt to measure the quality of nursing care delivered. The two are inextricably linked, since it is inevitable that the number of nurses and skills they possess will inevitably affect the quality of care received by the patient. The qualitative tools are discussed in more detail below.

Standard-based audit tools

Another option open to nurses wishing to measure the effectiveness of their care at a local level is the development of audit tools to measure the standards they have set. Methods for attempting to monitor care in this way are given below, with accompanying practical examples.

Criteria audits

Criteria-based audits can offer a quick, specific method for clinical nurses to gather data in an area of interest. Examples of how criteria-based audits can be used in practice are detailed later.

It became clear there were a number of options open to us when it came to auditing our nursing care. There were also a number of increasingly pressing reasons why we should attempt to perform an audit. Driven by these factors, we tried a number of different approaches in an attempt to audit our care; the practical applications of these varying approaches are included below.

Outlining practical application of various audit approaches

Undertaking a piece of research can be a useful learning experience, and we both found that working through the research process was of value in auditing care at a local level.

As part of the fourth year of the BSc Nursing Course we

were required to complete a 15,000 word dissertation. Initially this appeared a daunting task, however, after discussing our ideas with our respective supervisors and devising a plan with a timescale, the whole process felt much more straightforward. In carrying out the research, certain factors make the pathway much easier. First, as a researcher, you need to have clear ideas about which research methods you are going to use; this is where a supervisor is invaluable. The supervisor needs to direct the researcher's thinking without being prescriptive, so that ideas can develop and research does not stray onto the wrong path. It is an advantage if the supervisor insists on deadlines, as this ensures that the researcher paces their work, and does not try to complete any part of the research in a hurry. Meeting with the supervisor every two weeks maintains motivation and prevents unnecessary work that may not be of value to the research.

Small research grants may be available and it is worth contacting the RCN or your Regional Research Group/Nurse, who will be able to tell you of locally organized research schemes. Often you may only need funding for stationery, computer advice, postage, or library searches and articles. However, the cost of these can be quite high by the end of the project.

We also found that our managers were of immense support to us, as they understood the pressures of both working and studying and offered time to discuss problems and ways of solving problems that arose.

When you arrive at the point where you are ready to analyse results, the help of a computer expert will be extremely useful. Analysing vast amounts of data is not only time-consuming but tiring, especially if you possess only basic statistical analysis skills. Receiving advice from someone who can reduce manual tabulation and mental fatigue is one of the greatest helps to your project.

Problems will occur, however, and, prior to starting your project, establishing realistic timescales is an activity worth bearing in mind. Often you do not realize how long it is going to take you to complete interviews or transcribe the tapes, and this can add weeks to your timescale. Additionally, problems may arise when you want to conduct interviews, as the interviewees may be absent, on holiday or too busy to see you, which again delays your work.

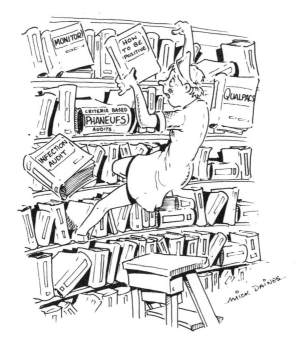

Illustration 2.1 Oh no! What will I choose?

The most important problem we came across was the length of time medical ethics committees took to grant permission for the research to be carried out. In some cases our colleagues experienced delays of up to 5 months before they received a decision. This is predominantly due to the committee being geared to medical rather than nursing research and the limited input professional nurses have on such committees.

Our experience of undertaking a research project helped us to identify key learning points which may be of use:

- Find a good supervisor, and plan your project in as much detail as possible.
- Make sure your research design is appropriate and always conduct a pilot study if using interviews, questionnaires or some form of a new instrument or tool.
- Ensure you have allowed sufficient time to write your project and to analyse any results.

- Share your results – this can be done at ward level, at unit level (by sending an information sheet to other wards and department) or by sending a synopsis of your work to one of the nursing journals.
- Take action on your findings – we both chose areas that were pertinent to our work at that time and therefore had an influence in improving the quality of care in our areas and influencing policy decisions for that area.

The advantages of using research, as opposed to other approaches, are that by choosing an area of interest, you are more motivated to complete the research and take action on the results. Furthermore, the research is geared to local needs and the findings are relevant to the local population. Carrying out a research project enhances many skills one would not necessarily utilize or learn elsewhere. These can include learning how to interview a person, formulating a questionnaire, performing a critique on a piece of work, synthesis of information and working to a timescale.

The disadvantages of using research to change practice is that the results tend to be too small to be significant or to draw general conclusions. They are not always transferrable to another area, as the field chosen can be too specific and take account only of local factors. Often, individuals within the area where the research is being conducted feel threatened about the research taking place, and this can affect the results obtained.

DATA COLLECTION AND PRESENTATION

When completing an audit and wishing to make changes to practice or policies, we have found that compiling a succinct report can be valuable in prompting or persuading other colleagues to recognize that the audit was of value. Part of preparing a report may be presenting data in one of the following ways:

- Simple graphs.
- Pie charts.
- Pictograms.
- Histograms.
- Bar graphs.

Simple graphs

If you wanted to demonstrate the trend of results from the Medical/Surgical Monitor (Goldstone et al., 1983) over the last 5 years, a simple graph (Figure 2.1) could be of use. Visually, this would appear more useful than writing each result for each year. Discussion of the reasons why the results peak and decline could then follow.

Pie charts

A pie chart is a circle divided into sections that correspond to the percentage of the item being depicted in the pie. For example, the percentage of the ward budget spent on continence supplies may be presented in this way (Figure 2.2). This information would make the reader aware of a number of interesting points. First, the large proportion of the budget spent on continence supplies may relate to:

- A large number of patients with continence problems being admitted to the ward.
- Inappropriate management of incontinence and a reliance on appliances and aids.
- Poor assessment and diagnosis, leading to poor management.

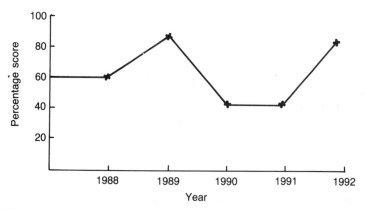

Figure 2.1 A simple graph showing results from the Medical/Surgical Monitor for the last 5 years.

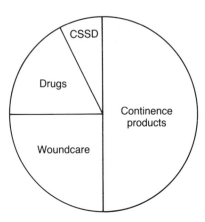

Figure 2.2 A pie chart showing the relative percentage of the ward budget spent on continence products.

Second, there may be a problem with the supplies of continence aids – perhaps an insufficient range of products to choose from, making nursing staff use whatever product is available, rather than the product most suitable for the patient. The pie should begin at 12 o'clock with the largest part of the pie. Following this clockwise, each successive segment should become smaller. This diagram could not be used to show spending over a number of months, but is useful for a particular event or month.

Pictograms

Pictograms offer the author a useful way of presenting data for a discussion or seminar. An example of this could be if you wanted to demonstrate to your nurse manager how ward study leave had decreased in the last four years and you felt this had a direct bearing on staff morale (Figure 2.3). The approach does not have to be light-hearted – you can choose how you wish to represent your data in any pictorial form.

Histograms

Pictorial or graphical representations of frequency or relative frequency are called histograms. A histogram should be self-explanatory and should allow the reader to identify relevant

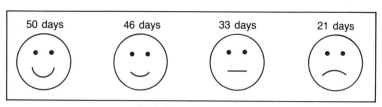

Study leave/staff morale

Figure 2.3 Pictogram showing the relationship between study leave and staff morale over the last 4 years.

aspects of the data. Each axis of the histogram should be labelled and each scale should be marked. An example could be the length of stay for patients who were admitted to the ward and the frequency of pressure sores developing, as illustrated below:

Length of stay	Frequency of pressure sores
5 days	1
10 days	2
15 days	4
20 days	7

A histogram could represent the above data as shown in Figure 2.4.

Bar charts

A bar chart is similar to a histogram except that the horizontal scale is a group of distinct categories or groups rather than continuous numerical intervals. An example is patients who present with continence problems relating to urge, stress or overflow incontinence (Figure 2.5).

In conclusion, you may find that presenting data in one of the above forms makes the reading of a report more enjoyable and more interesting. It condenses the information into a succinct and easily identifiable medium. Furthermore, it will have more impact on the reader than a page of writing.

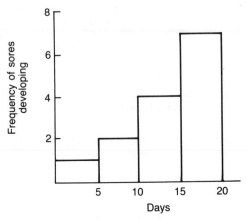

Figure 2.4 Histogram showing the relationship between length of stay in hospital and frequency of pressure sores.

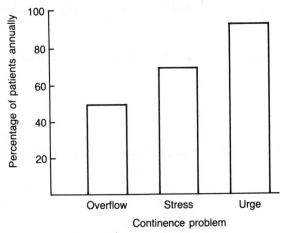

Figure 2.5 Bar chart showing the numbers of patients presenting with different continence problems.

OFF THE SHELF TOOLS

Monitor (Goldstone and Galvin, 1983)

Monitor is an audit tool used to indicate the quality of nursing care. It was first published by Goldstone and Galvin (1983) and is a reformatted version of the Rush Mediscus Audit system, which had been used in the USA. Following the widespread use of Medical/Surgical Monitor, subsequent versions relating to Paediatric Care (Goldstone and Galvin, 1983), Health Visiting (Goldstone and Whittaker, 1990), District Nursing (Goldstone and Illsley, 1989), Senior (Goldstone and Okai, 1989), Midwifery (Goldstone and Hughes, 1989) and Accident and Emergency (Goldstone, 1991) were developed.

The tool was devised to offer an index to quality (Goldstone and Illsley, 1985), i.e. a pointer, not a measure of quality. However, this principle has been misunderstood by a number of authors (Marsh and Brittle, 1986).

Monitor addressed the 'process' elements of nursing care. It also identifies the impact of laundry supplies, CSSD and domestic services on the ward. Monitor has been found to highlight deficiencies in care (Dickson, 1987) and in the care ethnic minorities receive whilst in hospital (Corrigan 1989). Many authors have questioned the validity of this tool (Barnett and Wainwright, 1987) mainly on the basis that an area with a high score may provide poor nursing care, and vice versa. This occurs because the majority of questions within this tool are based on documentation of care. Thus the assumption arises that what is documented is carried out, and to a standard that is acceptable. Also, staff are often now aware of the content of this audit tool and find it relatively easy to amend their documentation 2 days before the study in order to raise their score. Other authors highlight observer bias (Whelan, 1987). This should be eliminated in the training given to assessors, which should also ensure standard interpretation of the criteria. Assessors are also advised not to work in areas where they have close personal friends or have had previous difficulties with colleagues. However, there have been situations where assessors, appalled or surprised at low standards, have changed their behaviour and attitude accordingly (Corrigan, 1989). Fortunately, one can identify this during the assessment period on the ward, by frequent communication with the assessors or whilst analysing and interpreting the results.

The key to a successful audit is a comprehensive implementation plan and training of assessors in order to achieve valid results (Pullan and Chittock, 1986).

Some confusion is seen to exist in the underlying philosophy of Monitor because it is based on a nursing process framework yet claims to be applicable to task oriented nursing. However, it is feasible that staff who organize care using the task allocation can still use the nursing process to some degree and therefore this tool could still be used.

Guidelines for implementing a Monitor study

We have identified the following steps to take when implementing a Monitor study in practice:

- Ensure ward staff want to use the tool and understand how the study will be carried out and when.
- Type letters to patients giving informed consent, time and date of study.
- Train Monitor assessors, discussing issues such as their role, whether to wear uniform and name badges and what action to take should they come across an ethical situation they find difficult to handle. Training is usually implemented by organizing four 2-hourly sessions where the role of the assessor is fully explained in relation to impartiality and confidentiality. Advice is given relating to being an observer of a clinical practice or a situation they find difficult to deal with or unethical. An example of this may be finding a blood transfusion running through too quickly and no observations of the patient's pulse and temperature being taken. Assessors are advised to inform a nurse of their observations and record the action of the nurse. If they feel that no action was taken, the facilitator of the study will directly liaise with the nursing management of the ward and the assessor will have no further part in the event.
- Inform staff who the assessors are and prepare monitor books.
- Implement study.
- Analyse results and prepare a report. The results are fed into a computer, usually with the nurse in charge present. The facilitator and senior nurse identify good practice and areas that need improving. A balanced report is formulated explaining both.
- Feedback to ward staff. Feedback is given to staff by explaining both good and poor practice. Specific examples are given and the staff can question the results or request more information if they require it.

- Action plan – prepare with staff. Once all the staff are aware of the results, a meeting should be planned to facilitate the development of an action plan with as many staff as possible.
- Follow up the action plan. Re-evaluate progress.

Monitor's main weakness is that it relies very much on what is documented, and since its development in 1983, many of the criteria could now be described as redundant. Monitor has the potential to be a useful baseline tool and provide positive changes, depending on what happens after the audit. Having used this tool numerous times, we have experienced both positive and negative effects and outcomes. We have also seen colleagues counselled formally and ward staff become demotivated and resentful of the way in which the required changes were carried out, when little consultation took place and staff were told they had to change practice. Change management is therefore an essential factor.

A Case study outlining positive effects achieved using Monitor

A study was carried out on a 30-bed acute medical ward, which subsequently changed the way the ward was organized and greatly improved the quality of the service offered to patients. Although good practice was highlighted, the main problems following the study were identified as:

- Poor assessment of patients on admission.
- Medically oriented care plans.
- Poor evaluation of care plans.
- Lack of written information to patients.
- Poor clinical practice relating to:
  (i) Routine observations, e.g. unnecessary taking of temperature.
  (ii) Knowledge relating to a cardiac arrest, e.g. not knowing the procedure.
  (iii) Lifting and handling of patients, e.g. 'drag' lift up the bed.

With the full support of the manager, the ward staff devised their own action plan, which involved:

- A weekly ward meeting to discuss ward issues.
- All staff to undertake the Open University course 'A Systematic Approach to Nursing Care' (P 653).
- Development of a ward information leaflet.
- Reviewing the times and frequency of taking observations such as temperature, pulse and respirations.
- Review of lifting and handling practice for all staff on the ward.

All the recommendations outlined in the action plan were implemented within 6 months. This occurred because ward staff were involved from the early stages of planning the project and were not coerced by their manager into forcing change or implementing change at a pace that was unsuitable for the ward. Furthermore, the manager showed great support by attending all ward meetings and assisting wherever possible in facilitating the action plan, but not directing it.

Not all Monitor studies are carried out in this way with such positive results.

A Case study outlining negative effects achieved using Monitor

This study was carried out on a surgical unit where staff were told 'you will be monitored next month'. They did receive preparation regarding the study but had little choice regarding its implementation. The results of the study showed how:

- There were problems with assessment and evaluation of care.
- Patients complained of lack of sleep due to nurses talking loudly.
- Medications were omitted, and the reasons for this were not recorded.
- Clinical practice was poor in relation to:
  (i) Times of the administration of medication.
  (ii) Postoperative observations.
  (iii) Wound care, practice and policy.

Good practice was highlighted in many areas, however, and the staff recognized the problems identified and were willing to act on them with support.

Unfortunately they received no support from their manager and, after a 3-month period, it was evident that no changes had

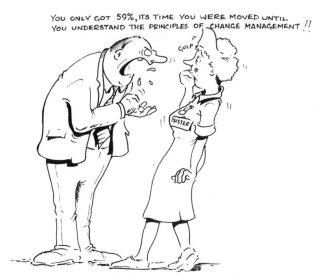

Illustration 2.2 You only got 59%

taken place. This was not surprising, for if the ward staff had understood how to facilitate the changes, they would have done so, but it was clear that they needed management support to facilitate continuing education needs. The senior Ward Sister was then formally counselled for failing to act on the findings of Monitor, and was removed from her post to another ward. No further action followed to improve the quality of care on this ward. The result was a demotivated workforce who felt quality assurance was simply a tool to beat staff when they did not fulfil the criteria.

Qualpacs audit

Qualpacs – Quality Patient Care Scales – was devised by Wandelt and Ager (1974), in the USA. Many of the criteria were derived from the Slater Nursing Performance Rating Scale (Slater, 1976), which audited the competence of the nurse giving the care.

Qualpacs – is classed as a concurrent tool in that it audits the quality of care of the patient on the ward.

Similar to Monitor (Goldstone and Galvin, 1983), Qualpacs reviews the patients' records and uses patient and staff interviews and observation of patients and observation of staff. It is divided into six categories with a total of 68 criteria:

- Physical   15 criteria.
- General   15 criteria.
- Communication   8 criteria.
- Psychosocial individual   15 criteria.
- Psychosocial group   8 criteria.
- Professional implications   7 criteria.

Following each criterion are instructions that tell the auditor that the observation is direct (D) or indirect (I). The scoring time for this tool is approximately 4 hours, which is similar to the scoring time for tools such as Senior Monitor. The auditors are advised to intervene if the patient is at risk.

Prior to carrying out direct observation, the auditor develops a plan of care for the patients based on the information available, and then observes the patient and listens for approximately 2 hours. When a nursing action is implemented the observer scores the item. For example, one of the criteria is 'The "rejecting" or "demanding" patient continues to receive acceptance', and this is rated as either Best Care, Between, Average Care, Between, Poorest Care, or Not Applicable or Not Observed. The weighting for each of these ranges from 5 to 1, with 'not applicable' or 'not observed' not scoring at all.

Whilst carrying out this audit, the observer can identify the carer. If a criterion is not observed, the auditor can look in the care plan for evidence of it being carried out.

After the items have been scored, the mean for each criterion is determined. These are then totalled and divided by the number of criteria scored.

Qualpacs has the advantage of observing the verbal and non-verbal behaviours of patients, nurses, carers, and other members of the multidisciplinary team. Furthermore, it uses more than direct observation to gain information and achieve a full picture of what is happening on the ward. As this tool is currently being evaluated in this country, and has been tested extensively in North America, it appears to have overcome the main problems displayed by audit tools such as Monitor (Goldstone and Galvin, 1983) and Phaneufs, i.e. over-emphasis on documentation and the nursing process. However, Qualpacs is time-consuming and has a complicated scoring system. We find it can be useful to ignore the scoring system in any audit tool and simply discuss the issues identified, not the scores. One could argue that auditors of Qualpacs may be subject to observer bias and that the scoring can be very subjective. Observers may allow their own personal feelings to enter into a situation and score more negatives or more positives depending on the situation.

Users of Qualpacs (Wainwright and Burnip, 1983) felt that some of the criteria are oriented towards the American pattern of nursing but also felt that many others were transferable to the British system of nursing.

Qualpacs is a valuable tool, which may need developing to suit British needs. However, it certainly highlights the value of auditing important nursing skills rather than just documentation of care.

Phaneuf's audit (1976)

This audit is a retrospective appraisal of the nursing process by reviewing the patient's notes – following discharge of the patient the nursing kardex and care plan are audited. The tool is therefore based on the assumption that all nursing care administered is accurately documented. In our experience this has proved to be a false assumption. Nurses often write a care plan according to the patient's medical diagnosis rather than their individual needs and ability to meet the actions prescribed on a care plan.

The audit was devised around the following topics:

- Reporting and recording care.
- Observations of symptoms and reactions.
- Supervision of patients.
- Implementation of nursing procedures.
- Health promotion via direction and teaching.
- The implementation of medical orders.
- Suppression of those participating in care.

It was suggested by the authors of the instrument that approximately five people audit up to ten records monthly post-discharge, and that the maximum time involved would be 15 minutes.

The tool consists of six or seven questions per topic, totalling

50 questions that need to be answered for each patient's record. Like most audit tools the tick boxes are 'yes', or 'no' or 'uncertain'. The last is present for use by the auditor if he/she feels the criteria have not been fully met. There is also a 'not applicable' box for the categories relating to nursing procedures and health promotion. The scores are totalled for all the components. Each of the 'yes' boxes has a predetermined weighted score. For example, in relation to the topic of physician/medical orders, if the medical diagnosis is complete and recorded accurately the score is 7. However, within the 'supervision of patient' category, if the nursing care plan has changed in accordance with the assessment of the patient the score is 4.

Having totalled all the scores in each section the quality of care is considered 'excellent' if the scores are 161–200; 'good' if between 121 and 160; 'incomplete' if between 81 and 120 and 'poor' if between 41 and 80. Less than 40 is considered 'unsafe'.

Phaneuf's audit is a simple tool, which is easy to implement and easy to understand. However, there are questions regarding its validity and efficiency. Although most areas utilize the nursing process to some degree, the tool relies heavily on documentation of care. Not all areas will find the questions applicable as the nursing process has been interpreted to suit a particular area. Therefore, many areas would 'fail' a question because staff verbally communicate some information, or presume knowledge or actions and would not record all such details in a care plan or kardex. An example of this would be the criteria relating to whether a patient has recreational or diversional activities recorded. This would be considered on a daily basis depending on the needs and wishes of the patient but would not necessarily be recorded in the care plan.

By carrying out this audit one measures the quality of nursing documentation rather than the quality of care. This tool was developed in North America and therefore many of the criteria relate to the health care system of America.

Advantages of using off-the-shelf tools

Off the shelf tools are easy to use as they have already been developed, tried and tested and are therefore ready for immediate use. The development of an audit tool can be a long process requiring a great deal of time in order to perfect it. The tools mentioned above give a broad picture of a ward predominantly using criteria-based tools on the nursing process format. They also act as a baseline measure over time and, given that the study could be carried out annually within the same framework, it should act as a reliable indicator of change in care standards. Therefore, these tools are replicable in the same and in different areas.

The above-mentioned tools require assessors who may be a staff nurse or the nurse in charge and can therefore find this a valuable learning experience.

As the tools are easy to implement, the data collected can be collated on software without difficulty.

Disadvantages of using off-the-shelf tools

Off the shelf tools generally tend to focus on documentation, although Qualpacs does depend more on observational skills. The focus of the tools tends to be non-specific, as they cover a wide range of topics and criteria. Areas that choose to undertake a study often feel anxious and threatened by having assessors – usually known to them – observing and checking documentation over a number of days. Regardless of preparation, most staff still admit to feeling nervous about these types of study.

CRITERIA-BASED AUDITS

A case study outlining the role of audit in improving infection control practices on a ward

Audits can also be carried out in response to an identified problem. On one particular ward of 34 elderly patients, a staff nurse felt that infection control procedures were being ignored. Although the hospital had no system for collating data on what type of infections occurred and where, staff on this particular ward observed a high incidence of catheter infections and occasional outbreaks of diarrhoea. In response to this, it was essential that data were collected to indicate the current problems relating to research and control of infection, and finally, the suggested outcome would be education of all staff in infection control practices.

The staff nurse (Horner, 1991) first observed all the staff on the ward during the course of her work and devised a simple audit tool that she could use to record whether practices were carried out. She then gave the staff nurses the audit questionnaire and asked them to identify their actions in response to control of infection. Examples of the criteria used are listed below:

- How often do you clean a patient's mattress and with what?
- When do you change oxygen tubing?
- How often do you clean your personal nursing scissors?

The audit results demonstrated that staff knowledge was poor in relation to research and infection control. Staff also thought that they carried out good practice when observation showed that this was not the case. An educational package was devised based on research articles, and teaching sessions were held every afternoon to disseminate information relating to good practice. Three months later the audit was carried out again. This time the practices relating to controlling infection had improved noticeably. The issues that had proved a problem were:

- Staff not washing their hands before serving meals.
- Staff being unaware of what 'good' research practice was in relation to catheter care.
- Gloves and aprons not being available in the sluice.
- Commodes not being cleaned after patient use.

All of the above have an impact on cross-infection and quality of care. No patient would be satisfied with their care if they received an infection that could have been avoided.

This particular audit proved two things. First, people at the 'grass-roots' level are concerned about their quality of work, and, second, they have the potential to do something about it if they are supported. The support must come from people who are able to facilitate their development but not control it.

Very often staff know the problems in their area only too well, but need guidance to resolve them. This applies particularly in a large organization where there are many people to contact, policies to adhere to and committees where issues can be raised. It is therefore of the utmost importance that there are mechanisms already in place so that staff know who to approach and can recognize that assistance will be available to help solve the problems.

A case study outlining the role of audit in evaluating a nursing innovation

Audits can also arise out of the need to explore a topic or because innovation in practice demands evaluation. Therefore issues raised through quality assurance are often very closely linked to research.

A self-medication audit arose in response to staff working on a ward caring for elderly people who wanted to review the quality of care given to patients. It was identified that elderly patients had all their drugs administered by nurses, in spite of the fact that the majority, when discharged, would have to take medication unaided. This conflicted with the values under-pinning Primary Nurse (i.e. that of partnership with one's patients and with the philosophy of the ward, i.e. the right of patients to make choices) and the aims of good nursing practice. One nurse decided to undertake a project to review why self-medication did not occur on this ward (Raycroft, 1991).

A questionnaire was given to all nurses in the ward with the aim of discovering information relating to the following criteria:

- What benefits there are from implementing a self-medication programme.
- What difficulties may arise.
- When and how should patients be assessed for taking their own medication.
- Where medication should be stored.
- Staff worries and fears relating to this programme.

Patients were given a questionnaire to complete. Those unable to do so were interviewed.

The results indicated that the majority of nurses: (i) were unaware of the hospital policy; (ii) did not know how self-medication would be organized; and (iii) felt unsure about the storage of medication.

Following publication of the results, the next stage was to ensure all staff knew the policy and were aware of how self-medication would be organized on the ward. A standard was set to enable all patients to be self-medicating. Criteria were set for safety relating to the storage of drugs. An example of the criteria within the standard were:

- The assessment of patients for the self-medication pro-gramme will be carried out by the Primary/Associate Nurse and involve the Pharmacist and medical staff.
- The care plan will clearly state lack of knowledge about medication and indicate patients' progress in the evaluation section.

Practice therefore changed as a result of carrying out a simple audit and following through the cycle for change. All members of the ward were involved and it was agreed to reaudit the project after 9 months (Figure 2.6). It was felt that the reason for success was because the action plan was generated by ward staff.

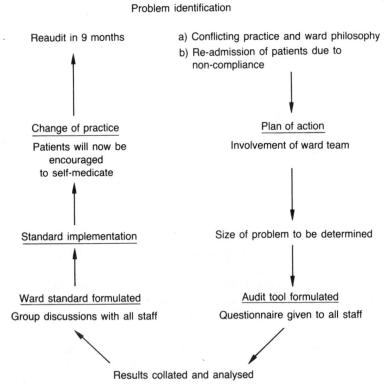

Problem identification

Reaudit in 9 months

a) Conflicting practice and ward philosophy
b) Re-admission of patients due to non-compliance

Change of practice

Patients will now be encouraged to self-medicate

Plan of action

Involvement of ward team

Standard implementation

Size of problem to be determined

Ward standard formulated

Group discussions with all staff

Audit tool formulated

Questionnaire given to all staff

Results collated and analysed

Figure 2.6 Cycle of change using criteria-based audits.

Patients admitted to the elderly unit now have control over their own medication and it is felt to be less likely that patients will be readmitted due to problems relating to non-compliance of medication. This is currently being audited by staff within the community, and by observing the readmission rate due to non-compliance of medication.

Advantages of criteria-based audits

We feel that criteria-based audits are a useful method for tackling a problem that staff feel might exist, but are unsure as to the scale of the problem, or the reason for its existence.

Valid, comprehensive and easy-to-audit criteria are formulated after study of research-based information, reading other audit tools and formulating questionnaires.

Staff at ward level are fully included in the whole change process and therefore feel less threatened by the audit. It also assists in the implementation of the action plan.

Disadvantages of criteria-based audits

The methods used to formulate a criteria-based audit are not methodologically pure and one could argue that the results obtained can only be specific for that area. If they were to be transferable, the tool would need to be piloted further and tested by a number of assessors to prove its validity. Only by having a very clear idea of what you are trying to measure will they be of use and avoid the trap of being general and non-specific.

STANDARD-BASED AUDIT TOOLS

When we discuss the structure, process or outcome criteria in nursing or the NHS we tend to place aspects of the organization into one of these criteria. For example:

- *Structure*, refers to the physical setting, the structure of the organization, financial aspects, objectives, buildings, equipment, attitudes of staff, etc.
- *Process*, refers to the actions taken by a nurse or member of staff or the care received by a patient.

- *Outcomes*, this would be the modification of symptoms of illness, knowledge, satisfaction, skill level, compliance with treatment. 'Outcome criteria consists of assessment of the end results of care usually specified in terms of patient health, welfare and satisfaction' (Donabedian, 1976). Donabedian's (1976) framework is discussed in more detail in Chapter 1.

For example, the criteria of structure, process and outcome as illustrated relating to pressure area care may be used as follows:

- *Structure*:
  (i)   RGN or EN;
  (ii) procedure number '1' pressure area care;
  (iii) pressure sore prevention protocol and research rationales;
  (iv) aids for pressure prevention, with manufacturer's manual;
  (v)   pressure sore audit forms.
- *Process*:
  (i)   each Primary Nurse (PN) or Associate Nurse (AN) will assess all patients on admission using the Waterlow score;
  (ii) all patients with a score of above 14 are identified as being at risk and problems, goals and nursing actions are identified;
  (iii) the PN or AN evaluates the effectiveness of the care plan;
  (iv) the PN or AN uses preventive aids according to protocol;
  (v)   the PN or AN attends in-service training on pressure sore prevention within 1 week of starting on the ward.
- *Outcome*:
  (i)   the incidence of patients developing pressure sores after admission is reduced to below 5%;
  (ii) nurses' knowledge of pressure sore prevention will increase to a score of >90% as indicated by educational score test results following in-service training;
  (iii) all patients at risk will have a legible, written plan of care.

Following the use of structure, process and outcome criteria developed for pressure area care, an audit tool can be developed (Table 2.1).

Table 2.1 Audit – pressure area care

Structure	Source	Yes/No	Exemptions
1. Does an RN or EN administer the patients pressure area care?	Observe		
2. Is the procedure No. 1 'Pressure Area Care' available on the ward?	Check records		
3. Is the protocol for Pressure Sore Prevention available on the ward?	Check records		
4. Are aids for pressure sore prevention in full working order?	Observe Ask nurse		
5. Do the nurses use the aids as outlined in manufacturers manual?	Observe		
6. Are Pressure Sore Audit forms available on the ward?	Check records		
Process			
8. If the Waterlow Scale is >14 does the patient have a problem, goal and nursing action documented within 6 hours of admission?	Check records		
9. Is this problem evaluated on every shift.'	Check records		
10. Does the nurse administer the care as prescribed?	Observe		
11. Is the Pressure Sore Audit Form completed and given to Senior Nurse following discharge?	Check records		
Outcome			
12. Does the nurse attend in service training sessions on pressure sore prevention within 1 week of starting on the ward?	Ask nurses		
13. Does the nurse achieve >90% in the post educational test?	Check records		
14. Are the plans legible?	Check records		
15. Is the annual incidence of pressure sores below 5%?	Check records		

Advantages of standard-based audit tools

The advantages of using standard-based audit tools are that the ward staff 'own' these standards and are therefore more likely to accept the standards as opposed to standards being imposed.

The standard audits will also reflect local needs and indeed change practice within that specific area or may be transferable to other areas with only slight changes. Audits of this nature are a natural progression from the formulation of standards and therefore assist staff in developing ideas of what can be suitably measured and what cannot.

It may also be possible to use outcome criteria when looking at clinical indicators for nursing. For example, if one was to assess the rate of pressure sores, or hospital-acquired infections, one may find within the outcome criteria that staff have insufficient knowledge to prevent such problems. In this situation, the outcome elements can be improved with limited resource implications.

Disadvantages of standard-based audit tools

There are a few problems associated with this method of auditing. The use of structure criteria can prove problematic because nurses often have little control over many of these variables where deficiencies are identified. There is also a danger in assuming that good care is ensured if all the necessary structure and process criteria are 'met. For example, instances where wards can be fully staffed, yet patients do not receive information regarding their illness and treatment. Thus one cannot attribute a link between structure and process and, furthermore, no evidence exists to suggest links between process and outcome. Measuring only outcome criteria can be a problem for the following reasons:

- General outcomes should not be used as a single indicator of quality because patients may have a positive outcome in spite of the care received, and not because of it.
- If staff feel that a patient must achieve a positive outcome within a specified period of time, they may well persuade a patient to achieve a goal at the expense of the holistic needs of the individual.

- It is difficult to discern if a nurse is solely responsible for a positive patient outcome because the involvement of the multidisciplinary team and the patient's own response to treatment can also influence the achievement of outcome measures.
- The lack of research into predicting patient outcomes as a result of direct nursing intervention makes it difficult for the nursing profession confidently to identify achievable outcome measures. Studies into medical practices attempting to link structure and process criteria with an identifiable outcome, show either no or limited correlation between the three variables.
- It is possible that close members of the patient's family, friends, or patients themselves, are other variables that influence the recovery.

Some authors suggest reviewing the goals set with the eventual outcome. In this way, sole use of any outcome can be avoided, giving nurses the opportunity to reflect on other components essential for patient care. However this approach assumes that nurses have the ability and confidence to set realistic goals and that the nursing process is used effectively by nursing staff. Research into the use of the nursing process by the profession does not support this assumption.

An answer to the above problems depends on support for practitioners from nurse education and nursing research. Research is required to develop standards of care and then predict reliable outcomes for specific patient groups, in response to a given nursing intervention. Nurses require further education and knowledge in order to formulate effective goals with patients. A first step to achieving this can be in the use of reflective practice. We have found that a useful method of encouraging this is to photocopy care plans for a small group of patients who have been discharged in the last month. The next step is to spend time with the primary or associate nurses discussing what the outcomes were in relation to the goals set. This may only take 1–1½ hours per month but assists nurses in thinking about the goals that they set.

Another useful exercise is for nurses to summarize the progress of a patient with members of the multidisciplinary team for specific groups of patients in an effort to review the overall success of multidisciplinary interventions. In this way, deficiencies in practice, lack of knowledge or the need for further research are identified. For example, the multidisciplinary team may find that during the last year 25% of patients who suffered cerebrovascular accident also developed limb contractions. There is a need to establish whether this is as a result of nursing knowledge relating to poor positioning, whether this is acceptable given the severity of strokes or conditions in which the client was admitted or if massage would have prevented such a problem occurring. What is important is the analysis of why the contractions developed and that standards were set and audited that demonstrate whether the process of care was effective.

The above approach is not without problems. For example, Table 2.2 shows a care plan of a patient with a sacral sore causing pain. Even if the nurse ensures an improved nutritional status, suitable wound care products, no pain and no pressure

Table 2.2 Patient care plan – sacral score

Date	Patient problem	Goal	Nursing action
	Jack feels his sacral sore is causing pain. Size of sore 4 cm × 4 cm Colour–yellow/ Green Depth <0.5 cm Waterlow Score–18	Reduce pain to <3 on pain scale	Offer prescribed analgesia ½ hour prior to treatment, dose according to severity of pain
		Reduce size to 1cm × 1 cm within 10 days	Clean area with normal saline, apply Scherisorb to sloughy area, apply occlusive dressing, review treatment every 4–7 days
			Ask Jack to alter position in bed 2-hourly
			Use Nimbus Mattress and pump
			Assess nutritional state– liaise with dietitian

applied to the sacral sore, one cannot be certain that the sore will be 1 cm × 1 cm in 10 days, or that this patient has the individual capacity for recovery.

Research has not proved conclusively that a combination of the above factors guarantees a predicted rate of wound healing. However, professional experience, gained as a result of caring for wounds, may allow the nurse to predict that the expected recovery rate should be 1 cm × 1 cm for the wound. Regrettably, nurses often fail to write case studies, reports or share information of such expertise to allow others to benefit from their experience.

AUDITING PRACTICE WITHIN A NURSING DEVELOPMENT UNIT

A Nursing Development Unit (NDU) is a care setting that aims to achieve and promote innovation and excellence in nursing practice in a hospital, neighbourhood or health authority. NDUs experiment in good practice, supported by research, management and education. The climate they seek to create is one where change in practice and questioning of practice is seen as part of the normal nursing culture.

In order to establish an NDU one would normally seek criteria from the Kings Fund or from one's Regional Department of Nursing, depending on local difference. These criteria involve determining leadership, defining specific projects, evaluation techniques, financial proposals, the current philosophy and management support.

Establishing an NDU on a secure foundation is a complex process, and we found that as the funded development units were just beginning, it was difficult to find other nurses who were in the same situation. However, we both felt that, with or without funding, innovation in practice could be implemented and the quality of care improved in an elderly care setting. Very often, nurses fail to realize how much change they have succeeded in initiating over a period of time and we felt recognition for such hard work should be made.

The philosophies in both our NDUs were different, as they reflected the values and beliefs of staff in that particular area. However, the staff of both units felt they were willing to try and change any aspect of practice if improvements in patient care could be made.

Auditing Nursing Development Units

Auditing the major and rapid changes which take place when starting an NDU is a difficult and demanding undertaking. Many facets associated with the staff's philosophical beliefs, nursing practice, the organizational structures, management and individual staff development, are affected by the decision that a ward or group of wards wish to develop nursing practice.

The recipients of change are not only the patient, the nursing staff and other members of the multidisciplinary team, but those outside that particular area, such as the budget-holder, other areas of nursing and charitable groups and organizations outside the National Health Service.

Thus, to audit an NDU one is seeking to measure both internal and external effects. This can be achieved in a number of ways, and the framework outlined below is simply one way of achieving this, and will in fact depend upon the aims and objectives that are to be implemented. However, the eclectic approach outlined may indeed be of use to many staff seeking to audit change within an NDU.

Depending on the aims and objectives originally developed, it is feasible to audit the changes that occur by looking at what has been achieved through your action plan. For example, one of the aims of the NDU in which we worked stated that 'Care planning would eventually be collaborative with the multi-disciplinary team'. A year later, it was easy to audit this. The most difficult changes to audit are those relating to beliefs and attitudes of the staff; these require a more in-depth research study.

There are many reasons for wanting to audit change within an NDU. First, one has to justify the cost if a grant has been given to fund the unit, particularly if it is for only one ward. Second, one has a professional duty to prove that the input of a facilitator or change agent whose function is to promote change, maintain the impetus for change and evaluate the change, is, in fact of benefit to staff and can produce more positive effects than the ward staff trying to fulfil this function alone. Some areas that have started an NDU specifically employ a person to act as a change agent without having managerial or hierarchical 'power'. The title for such a role may be Researcher, Advisor, Facilitator or Clinical Nurse Specialist.

They may work within one ward or a number of wards to move change forward.

Some sceptics of NDUs have voiced the opinion to us that changes in practice would happen automatically if a ward had a 3-year plan for development, whether the ward was called an NDU or not. This may well be true, although no thorough evaluation of any area has taken place to prove that such changes can occur without a facilitator moving the changes forward and without some extra source of funding being available for this to occur.

Auditing changes over the period of time from inception to fulfilment of goals must also be a valuable and worthwhile exercise for all staff. They receive recognition for their hard work, have a great input into deciding the future projects of the ward and fulfil personal objectives regarding patient care that they feel are important.

We personally believe that NDUs should not be restricted to one ward and can indeed operate successfully in a number of wards of the same speciality, thus having a 'unit'. This allows for the sharing of ideas, a greater sharing of resources and the reduction of elitism. Furthermore, when organizing in-service training, it is difficult to teach or facilitate groups when staff can only be released from one ward. Involving more than one ward solves this problem and also gives the ward staff the opportunity to mix with other wards and discuss ideas.

Problems of elitism can occur if one ward is singled out for development, particularly if given extra resources to initiate projects. If more than one ward participates the resources can be shared in a number of wards and the impact of a project spread to more than one area.

The need for audit is a reflection of management, professional and political necessities to ensure that NDUs are not a 'flash in the pan', but are the way forward for nursing to develop innovative practice.

Framework for auditing a Nursing Development Unit

All the tools listed below are of use not only to the nursing staff at ward level but to managers of the unit as well. Using a variety of tools can illustrate improvements in the quality of care, innovations in practice and staff development, and the effects of these practices on other areas within and outside the hospital can be seen. Efforts to establish the cost–benefits of improved practice are also a useful and effective way of demonstrating to managers why it is important to invest and indeed support those wishing to implement an NDU.

Whilst developing plans for an NDU baseline data can be obtained:

- Sickness and absence data.
- The presence of individual performance review.
- Amount of study time/leave.

The above data are of use when explaining to managers how increased staff appraisal, setting specific staff objectives, and having a systematic ward development plan can improve staff morale and improve staff attendance.

- Patient accident rates.
- Patient satisfaction with care and choice of service.
- Overall indicator of quality, e.g. Qualpacs, Monitor.

Evaluating patient accident rates can be of use when trying to improve safety for patients by determining if a particular area of the ward is more at risk than another and if steps need to be taken to specifically identify patients who can be more at risk than others. Accident rates may also indicate times of short staffing, if correlated to staff off duty, or may indicate that more attention needs to be paid to reducing restraint, e.g. use of cot sides, if this proves to be a cause of accidents.

Patient satisfaction questionnaires carried out on a monthly basis for a defined number of patients may show that, as practice changes, there is a corresponding rise of patients' satisfaction with care. However, this initiative should not be used alone but in conjunction with the overall quality of care indicator. Using a tool such as Qualpacs or Monitor can serve as a useful baseline tool as outlined previously.

- Number of staff projects.
- Utilization of nursing process (modified Brookings tool; Corrigan, 1990).

Identifying the current amount and type of staff projects will demonstrate if staff are currently developing research skills and feel confident to question practice and innovate new practice.

This information will assist in planning the educational requirements for the ward and the in-service training programme.
Identifying how effective nurses are in utilizing the nursing
process will assist in planning training needs, but will also
identify whether care is research-based, individualized and the
extent to which the patient is involved in their care. Having
completed baseline data, you may wish to proceed to tackle
specific problems and develop criteria-based audits depending
on the needs of your wards. Examples of these audits include
topics such as:

- Infection control (practice and rates).
- Use of self-medication (reasons why used/why not used).
- Type of wound products used (use and evaluating success).
- Amount of choice in diet for elderly patients.
- Back injury rates.
- Continence audit (practice based on research and rituals).

These audits can be implemented and a training/teaching
programme initiated to tackle the problem. The topic can be
reaudited and this would demonstrate a clear improvement in
practice. It is worth contacting other NDUs to find out if the
above criteria-based audits have already been formulated,
which will save time and effort on your behalf.

When the NDU has established itself and developments in
practice have taken place, staff may feel they want to review
the overall impact of the changes on the ward or unit. This can
be undertaken by reviewing the initial baseline data. However,
further evaluation tools may be utilized as listed below:

- Reduction in infection rates (length of stay, antibiotics).
- Reduction in length of stay, e.g. with improved discharge
  planning.
- Reduction in the cost of continence supplies.
- Number of articles published by the unit.
- Number of visitors and exchange programmes.
- Consultancy time spent with other health authorities.

Auditing the length of stay may show that improvements in the
implementation of a discharge policy reduces length of stay, or
even readmission rates, by ensuring that when patients are
discharged the multidisciplinary team works collaboratively
and potential problems are eliminated. Costs such as continence

supplies may be reduced because of an effective in-service training programme and more appropriate continence aids being used for patients (Watson, 1990).

The external influence of the impact of the NDU may be established by the number of visitors to the unit or the amount of time spent visiting other areas acting as a consultant or advisor.

The number of articles published could be an indicator of staff who are prepared to spend time writing about new practices or their experience with less well researched practices, such as primary nursing.

Some of the initiatives used in this framework are discussed later in detail (Chapter 3). Many other evaluation techniques may be used to demonstrate the effects of change to patients, to staff and to those outside an NDU, depending on your original aims and strategy for changing practice.

CONCLUSION

Many of the approaches to audit described above proved useful in beginning the process of changing and improving the quality of nursing care.

The main difficulty we experienced with this approach was that the whole audit process can quickly accelerate into an unplanned, uncoordinated number of initiatives. In practice, this created three key problems.

First, staff were developing and using audit tools without monitoring and supervision. In some instances, this led to a number of poorly designed tools being used and dubious data being produced. Staff had therefore invested significant time and effort in a project that had limited use. Without proper monitoring of such initiatives, there were also instances of duplication of effort, with several areas developing tools for similar projects, such as auditing nursing documentation and pressure area care management. It also meant that where good practice was identified, there was no mechanism for disseminating this to other areas.

Second, lack of co-ordination can lead to lack of co-operation from those participating in the audit because of being over-loaded with similar requests from different areas. This prompted one patient to ask whether it was possible to go to any department in the hospital without feeling obliged to participate in a patient satisfaction survey!

The final difficulty with focusing purely on audit was the lack of a systematic approach to resolving deficiencies in care identified through the audit process. Some areas went on to take action to rectify these. Some areas used the results in a punitive way, making staff hostile to future audits. There were also examples where re-auditing several months later identified exactly the same deficiencies in care.

It was identified that, although audit was an important factor in 'making quality happen', there were other factors that needed to be incorporated to ensure optimum value was obtained from the staff time invested in audit activities.

Chapter 3 will explore the use of well-validated audit tools available to nurses, and the use of frameworks to co-ordinate and monitor the cycle of quality improvement.

REFERENCES

Barnett, D. and Wainwright, P. (1987) Between two tools. *Senior Nurse*, **614**, 40–2.

Corrigan, P. (1989) *Evaluation of Monitor Project*. Seacroft/Killingbeck Hospitals.

Corrigan, P. (1991) *An Examination of the Extent to Which the Nursing Process is Implemented on Primary Nursing Ward in Comparison to a Team Nursing Ward*. BSc Thesis, Leeds Metropolitan University.

Dickson, N. (1987) Do you measure up? *Nursing Times*, **83** (44), 25.

Donabedian, A. (1976) *Some Issues in Evaluating the Quality of Health Care in Issues of Evaluation Research*. American Nurses Association.

Goldstone, L., Ball, J. and Collier, M. (1983) *Monitor – an index of the quality nursing services on acute medical and surgical wards*. Newcastle Upon Type Polytechnic Products, Newcastle Upon Tyne.

Goldstone, L. (1984) *Monitor – Medical – Surgical*. Newcastle Upon Tyne Polytechnic Products, Newcastle Upon Tyne.

Goldstone, L. (1991) *Accident and Emergency Monitor*. Newcastle Upon Tyne Polytechnic Products, Newcastle Upon Tyne.

Goldstone, L. and Galvin, J. (1983) *Paediatric Monitor*. Newcastle Upon Tyne Polytechnic Products, Newcastle Upon Tyne.

Goldstone, L. and Hughes, D. (1989) *Midwifery Monitor*. Newcastle Upon Tyne Polytechnic Products, Newcastle Upon Tyne.

Goldstone, L. and Illsley, V.A. (1985) *A Guide to Monitor*. Newcastle Upon Tyne Polytechnic Products, Newcastle Upon Tyne.

Goldstone, L. and Illsley, V.A. (1989) *District Nursing Monitor*. Newcastle Upon Tyne Polytechnic Products, Newcastle Upon Tyne.

Goldstone, L. and Okai, M. (1986) *Senior Monitor*. Newcastle Upon Tyne Polytechnic Products, Newcastle Upon Tyne.

Goldstone, L. and Whittaker, C. (1990) *Health Visiting Monitor*. Gale Centre Publications, Loughton.

Horner, P. (1991) *Infection Control Audit*. Medical Unit, United Leeds Teaching Hospitals Trust, Leeds.

Marsh, J. and Brittle, J. (1986) Monitor – definition of measurement. *Nursing Times*, **82**, 36–7.

Mayers, M. (1983) *A Systematic Approach to Nursing Care Plans*. Appleton, Century Crofts, New York.

Phaneufs, M. (1976) *The Nursing Audit*. Appleton Century Crofts, New York.

Polit, D.F. and Hungler, B.P. (1990) *Essentials of Nursing Research*. J.B. Lippincott, Philadelphia.

Pullan, B. and Chittock, C. (1986) Quantifying quality. *Nursing Times*, **January 1st**.

Raycroft, A. (1991) *An Investigation Into the Use of Self Medication on our Elderly Care Unit*. Medical Unit, United Leeds Teaching Hospitals Trust, Leeds.

Slater, C. (1989) An analysis of ambulatory care, quality assessment research. *Evaluation and the Health Profession*, **12** (4), 347–78.

Wainwright, P. and Burnip, S. (1983) Qualpacs at Burford. *Nursing Times*, **February 2nd**, 36–8.

Wandelt, M.A. and Ager, J. (1974) *Quality Patient Care Scales*. Appleton, Century Crofts, New York.

Watson, R. (1990) The concept of cost-effectiveness. *Nursing Standard*, **4** (31), 36.

Whelan, J. (1987) Using Monitor – observer bias. *Senior Nurse*, **7** (6).

3

Quality Assurance

The last two chapters explored some of the tools and techniques used in audit. However, audit is but one part of the cycle which aims to assure the quality of care or service. The term 'quality assurance' (QA) is often thought to encompass everything from counting every stock item in the hospital to discounting any arduous project as the responsibility of a newly appointed QA Manager. This has, not surprisingly, led to many misconceptions about the definition, purpose and function of a QA programme.

This chapter will examine the reasons why QA has become increasingly prominent within the NHS, and then describe some of the methods used in the effort to enhance quality of care. Donabedian (1966) notes that 'quality at best can be protected and enhanced but not assumed'.

Throughout, our personal experiences will be discussed in addition to the different methods used and, following this, the frameworks for QA will be discussed and critiqued.

HISTORY OF QUALITY ASSURANCE IN THE NHS

The use of QA programmes and initiatives has developed predominantly from the Griffiths Report (1983). The report postulated 'whether the NHS is meeting the needs of the patient and the community, and that it can prove so, is open to question'. It also made it clear that there are a number of groups the NHS should satisfy, and that these groups not only include patients, but NHS employees, the community and the tax-payer.

The idea of monitoring quality of care is not new. Florence Nightingale evaluated the care that was delivered to patients, and used the information to improve care in areas that were below standard (Harrison, 1958).

Despite the rapid growth of QA in industry, the development of similar methods in the NHS was very slow, and, within the nursing profession, little work took place. Authors such as Abdellah (1958) did some work in terms of multidisciplinary care conferences and the quality of care related to skill mix, but such studies attempting to monitor quality were in the minority.

By the 1960s the Salmon Report (1966) had a more direct effect on the nursing profession in terms of management skills and the efficiency of the service. Certainly, as the Royal College of Nursing developed, it became involved in standards of care and the development of the RCN Standards of Care Project (RCN, 1980). This Steering Committee then produced documents such as *Towards Standards* (RCN, 1981), which were then further developed by Kitson (1986).

Other bodies, such as the Community Health Councils, came into being in 1973, in order to give lay people a say in the management of hospitals and to give the consumer a voice. Voluntary organizations have also proved successful in the last 15 years in continuing the momentum of improving the quality of care. These include organizations such as NAWCH (National Association for the Welfare of Children in Hospital), Age Concern and MIND (National Association of Mental Health). The Charter for Children in Hospital, produced in 1984, has, in our experience, encouraged Nurse Managers to monitor the standards of care within Childrens' Departments. It has also provided an impetus for change in meeting these standards within a department. For example, they stipulate that no child under 15 years of age should be admitted to an adult ward, and efforts should be made to ensure that this does not happen. This standard has been adhered to in hospitals where we have worked.

How far International and National mandates affected the development of quality assurance is difficult to say. The World Health Organization stated that 'by 1990 all member states should have built effective mechanisms for ensuring quality of patient care within the health care system' (WHO, 1985). Although policies were developed by health authorities, these were not necessarily implemented. However, John Moore (1988), then the Secretary of State for Social Services, believed 'that we must ensure that the customer is not only consulted, but that his or her views are acted upon whenever possible'. It is fair to say that, within many health authorities, it was not until 1987 that a co-ordinated, planned effort was made to evaluate the quality of care or to address the concept of quality.

APPROACHES TO QUALITY ASSURANCE

The understanding of QA varies widely within the NHS. Some may believe that quality can be recognized, but a comprehensive definition has so far proved elusive.

The definition offered by the Collins English Dictionary is that quality is 'a grade of goodness or excellence'. This is a limiting definition, and Pursig (1974) notes that people differ about quality not because quality is different but because people are different in terms of experience.

Health authorities have adopted a diverse range of approaches in striving to fulfil directives imposed from Regional and Government services. The approach used can be a mixture of consumer focus and cost reduction. Thus there can be different motives for promoting quality within a health care setting. However, if quality becomes a political issue, as directed by Regional and District dictat, somewhere along the line the profession aims and expectations of quality assurance may be lost. One risk of losing professional commitment was evidenced in the USA when the Professional Standards Review Organization was formulated (WHO, 1985). This had the reverse effect of alienating professional groups instead of encouraging involvement in QA. Within the UK, most professional groups (nursing in particular), have made efforts to be involved in and to promote QA. Where this has failed to happen it may owe as much to the methods used by management to introduce quality initiatives, as to the professional groups themselves.

The approaches used have depended upon previously formulated conceptual models, industrialist approaches or focus on specific elements, e.g. measurement or quality circles.

Many approaches focused initially on measurement (Wysenewski, 1988), which is logically consistent with the competitive approach to QA. This approach assumes that once we have the kinds of measures of quality that enable customers to distinguish among different levels of quality, improvements and control will fall into place.

Some approaches have veered towards the industrialist methods. An example of this are the concepts, e.g. offered by Crosby (1979) where 'getting it right first time' should form the basis of a QA strategy. This has been adopted by QA managers, who have used these principles successfully in QA programmes (Blakelock, personal communication).

Morris (1989) feels the emphasis placed on routine evaluation of what has happened in the health service is of little benefit to patients experiencing problems of service. Not only that, but time, energy and materials that do not conform to existing standards are a waste. Thus, 'defining and agreeing requirements' is the first stage in the development of a QA strategy.

REASONS FOR PARTICIPATING IN QUALITY ASSURANCE PROGRAMMES

There are many reasons why health service professionals should become involved with quality assurance, even though this may mean added pressures at work or increased workload.

Professional reasons

Nurses are accountable for their actions and, professionally, we have a responsibility to evaluate the effectiveness of our care in the light of new research findings. An example of this would be that nurses no longer use egg white and oxygen on pressure sores, or leave wounds exposed to 'dry' out, because research findings have proved these practices ineffective for quality patient care. Most professionals also want to deliver a high standard of care, and being empowered to identify and resolve problems can add to personal satisfaction with work.

Social reasons

One can argue that, ethically, everyone has the right to the highest attainable level of health, a value the World Health Organization embraces. Furthermore, in health care the stakes are high and the life of a person may be at risk. Therefore, guaranteeing standards of care to the public must be a duty of all those who work within the health service. Documents such as the Patients' Charter (1992) state clearly how the health service should perform and what the patients can expect.

Political and economic reasons

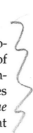

At a time when resources are scarce it is vital that health professionals, and nurses in particular, demonstrate the value of their contribution to the organization. Furthermore, the managerial emphasis from organizational and government schemes is for 'value for money', as evidenced by reports such as *Virtue of Patients* (1991) and the recent Value for Money document (1991).

Nursing has made a significant impact in developing quality assurance in the NHS. Dalley's (1989) work found that although general managers bear overall responsibility for QA, 20% of the designated officers throughout the service came from a nursing background. However, with the emphasis now being placed on the 'total quality management' approach, the trend towards general managers' overall accountability may well continue to develop.

Dalley's (1989) study also found that activities relating to QA were carried out by 38% of nurses, and that the second largest group to be involved were the paramedics (1989). The activities that nurses tend to be involved in are audit, service reviews, standard-setting and customer relations.

There would seem to be no doubt about the current interest in QA among British nurses, but whether it will continue as a specialized function, or become incorporated in normal day-to-day management is a question (raised by Glennester, 1986) that is still unanswered.

An area where some work has been carried out by nurses is in the application of performance indicators related to the process and outcome of care. Reid (1986) feels that performance indicators pose more questions than answers. However, Vetter (1986) applied performance indicators in the care of the elderly, as did Caddow (1986) in the field of infection control. Reid (1986) stresses that computerized performance indicators, such as the DHSS package relevant to clinical activity, can be useful analytical tools, but cannot be used in isolation from other information.

UK are also in a unique position of implement-
s, not because they have to but because they
Benner (1984) points out the advantage of this
o in the US, where nurses were forced to
_, assurance programmes through fear of law
suits, denial of accreditation and loss of revenue.

The current status of quality assurance as viewed by the nursing profession appears to focus on setting standards, auditing the process of nursing care and developing outcome measures, whilst looking simultaneously at wider issues, such as skill mix. Much work in this field has already been carried out by the Royal College of Nursing (RCN) (1981).

Standards such as Rheumatic Diseases were published by Royal College of Nursing, and other specialities are following. The framework is based on structure, process and outcome criteria. However, authors such as Williamson (1988) have used a more flexible system, which consists of standard statements with an attached score sheet for computer analysis, although many others, such as Sale (1988), are following the framework of structure, process and outcome. In psychiatric areas experimentation with frameworks is occurring as evidenced by the work of Blakelock (personal communication).

Another initiative widely adopted has been the use of quality circles, and these continue to be used in many areas as a method of improving quality. The use of quality circles and other methods used to improve the quality of patient care will now be discussed more fully.

THE USE AND SUCCESS OF QUALITY CIRCLES

Quality circles are a process whereby staff at every layer in an organization work together as a team using problem-solving techniques to improve quality of services and working life.

The process starts by:

- Identification of problems, which involves selecting a problem for study and exploring and agreeing on solutions.
- Presenting solutions to management, or implementing solutions if appropriate.
- Evaluation of problem and effectiveness of solutions.

Quality circles originated in the industrial sector of Japan and were pioneered by Deeming and Juran (Incomes Data Services Ltd, 1985). The concept spread to the health service sector by the early 1980s and was used extensively by North Warwickshire Health Authority (Hyde, 1984). Quality circles were set up to allow increased staff participation in management decisions as part of a new 'bottom up' approach by the authority. They were considered not as an entity in themselves, but as part of a new management philosophy.

Quality circles were found to change working practices, (Johnson and Clarke, 1984), and develop the team approach to care (Johnson, 1984). When used in the US by the nursing profession, communication increased by 80% on a ward, there was 60% increase in job satisfaction and 70% increase in morale.

Most articles can describe how to formulate a quality circle, but very few actually point out why some circles fail and others succeed. Davies (1985) does point out that there are difficulties in finding time for health care workers to meet on a multidisciplinary basis, and this may cause a lack of motivation. This leads to failure of the quality circle, but no examples are cited where this has occurred.

Quality circles (according to the study by Dalley (1989)) comprise 6.8% of all quality initiatives, and 46% are evaluated after use. The Royal College of Nursing *Quality Assurance Directory* of 1988 noted that quality circles were used by 17 health authorities in the UK. The areas in which quality circles were most commonly used were General Acute and Psychiatry.

Our views of quality circles are very much in keeping with Johnson (1984), in that they are of use providing the circle members (whatever their discipline) meet through their own choice and end the circle when problems have been solved. Advocates of quality circles often suggest that a circle should continue, as there are always issues and problems to solve. Our experience shows that quality circles pull people together within a team, give the opportunity to allow ideas to flourish and, most importantly, solve problems. We have found that within the nursing profession, quality circles have achieved the above in many areas and, furthermore, have moved a ward or department forward in new practice.

However, we have also seen motivated staff become demoralized when they have put a great deal of effort into finding information regarding a topic, planning changes only to find that a lack of support from management meant the solutions were never realized. In another example, the facilitator cancelled meetings and generally lacked commitment, and the circle failed.

Below we have described two quality circles – one that showed positive benefits and one that failed.

The positive benefits from a Quality circle

A group of ward-based nurses who worked on a 25-bed surgical unit using team nursing met to discuss problems identified on the ward. The ward was divided down the middle into two teams, 'A' and 'B'. Problems identified by the quality circle were:

- The large number of patients with catheter infections.
- Why some information did not get passed on to staff.
- The lack of co-ordination at a cardiac arrest.
- The uncertainty staff felt when dealing with patients who had problems with wounds.

The staff decided to tackle the issue of communication and information that somehow 'got lost'. They brain-stormed all the issues that related to this aspect and the following were high-lighted:

- Reports were too long and not very specific.
- Care plans were not up to date.
- Care plans were not in use.
- The person 'in charge' sometimes forgot to communicate information.
- Staff did not know which information to write on the care plan and which on the communication sheet.
- Some staff felt that if care plans were kept by the patient's bed they would be of more use.

What became evident was that the ward was divided, not just in its views relating to 'communication' but philosophically in its values relating to nursing and patient care. Other themes to emerge include:

- Should patients have access to their nursing care plans and assessment?

- Should patients share in the assessment and care planning stages?
- Should reports include the patient?

Tackling the issues relating to the above opened the proverbial 'can of worms'. The solutions sought to each of the problems identified included:

- A short report should take place in the office for all staff to give information relating only to severely ill patients, patients undergoing investigations and any other significant information.
- Following this, the nurses on the earlier shift would give a direct handover to the nurses on the following shift for that particular team, i.e. 'A' or 'B'.
- Staff felt that they needed to discuss the importance of care planning and access to notes with patients, and agreed as a team how this should be carried out.
- Agreement on the importance of including the patient in all stages of assessment, planning, evaluation and, most importantly, the 'implementation' stage.
- Asking the person in charge to have two wipe boards in the office so that important messages could be written down for the next group of staff.

All of the above required the Ward Manager to be open to change, respect the views of staff and implement the solutions that were finalized. It required open discussions with all staff valuing the opinions of other members regardless of their place in the nursing hierarchy.

Luckily, the facilitator dealt with many of these issues in the first meeting and, although the ward manager was asked if she would like to start a quality circle, the impetus for change following this came from the team as a whole. Thus, no pressure or coercive tactics were necessary for the development of solutions.

The staff on this ward implemented the solutions to the problems and went on to tackle the other issues identified; this took 18 months to complete. However, the learning experience and the success of the change was internalized into the ward culture.

The negative effects of Quality circles

A group of nursing staff on a 34-bed acute medical ward met with a trained facilitator to discuss the problem of the lack of patient/relative information. Their problem was that they wanted to include information relating to how the nurses cared for patients but were unsure how to do so. They also wanted it to be in large print and have an eyecatching design.

The group met in total three times. The first time they set their ground rules, discussed the remit of the group and discussed the problem at length.

The second time they 'brain-stormed' ideas of how they could go about providing this information. This included:

- A friend of one of the staff designing the art work.
- A group working on the content of the booklet.
- One nurse finding out if this idea was acceptable to the manager and in keeping with the organization's documentation.

The final time the group met all the above information had been gathered and the final plans were to be agreed.

The facilitator of the group had the resources to print the documentations, and offered to do this. Usually a 'facilitator'

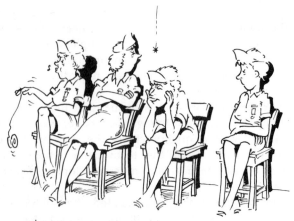

WELL! WE'VE ALL THE TIME IN THE WORLD TO WAIT FOR THE FACILITATOR HAVEN'T WE?

Illustration 3.1 Waiting for the facilitator.

keeps to the remit of their role, i.e. to move the group forward but not to be involved directly in the solutions. However, this time the remit changed due to the facillitator's position in the organization.

The fourth meeting, which should have detailed the cost of the printing and the date for this to take place, never actually took place. The facilitator cancelled the meeting due to other commitments and although the circle repeatedly contacted her to arrange another meeting none was forthcoming. This caused the staff to feel demoralized, after all the work they had undertaken, and also to view quality circles in a negative light. The group should, in our opinion, have sought their own solutions to the printing issue. However, the facilitator had become an important part of the group, and not just the 'facilitator' of the group, and no other leader emerged to resolve these issues.

This experience highlights that it is essential that all who participate in quality circles understand what they involve, and the time element, in order for the quality circle to succeed.

CUSTOMER SATISFACTION SURVEYS

Users of the NHS cannot select the hospital doctor or nurse of their choice. However, it is clearly important to enable patients to indicate where the service can be improved.

Patient studies, or satisfaction surveys, have been around for a long time. As early as 1957, in the US, Abdellah and Levine sought to establish patients' views. A similar British study was carried out by McGhee in 1961 and another, later, by Cartwright (1964).

Work by Raphael (1967) led to the development of King's Fund questionnaire, which was then modified by Raphael (1969). Nehring and Geach (1973) question the value of patient satisfaction questionnaires because of the 'halo' effect. They feel that patients would be reluctant to criticize nurses if they were going to be in hospital a long time or have readmissions. Ventura (1982) reports that high levels of satisfaction with nursing care are due also to the 'halo' effect.

A study carried out by UMIST with the Community Health Councils in 1982 developed a questionnaire which in their view 'was sufficiently detailed to solicit responses which could be used to bring about improvements' (Moores and Thompson, 1985). In all, 1357 usable questionnaires were returned from seven different hospitals. From this, six underlying dimensions of 'patient satisfaction' were elicited, most of which applied to the 'structure and process' variables, although these were not listed in the study for reference.

Although many Health Authorities have since commissioned studies of this size, other Health Authorities, such as Bloomsbury, have chosen 12 questions to ask patients as part of routine monitoring. The project, funded partly by the Department of Health, was to grant the 'clinical accountability service planning and evaluation' project (CASPE) money to develop a methodology to monitor patients' views routinely, and use a computer-readable system to analyse the results. The Government has an interest in this area, as can be seen by the prescription of routine use of surveys to monitor patient satisfaction within the NHS and self-governing hospitals (White Paper, 1989). The White Paper also implies that managers should be able to assess, interpret and respond to changes in the level of satisfaction.

Critics of this method feel that specific disquiet amongst patients will be over-ruled by global satisfaction (Carr-Hill, 1989). Also, as the respondents have a choice of 'very satisfied', to 'very dissatisfied', any other response is ruled out, and so the responses fall into narrow bands. The tool is thought to be too formal to provide valid or detailed information.

According to Carr-Hill (1989) simple questions are relatively insensitive. However, Crown (1989) feels that it is a cost-effective sampling method which has brought about many changes and resulted in an improved service. Questions still arise, however, as to the way the surveys are administered by hospital staff, especially when the respondents are still captive within an institutional environment, and the effect this may have on the results. It is also questionable whether such substantial investment is needed in order to ascertain if the food is of poor quality and inedible.

Despite the difficulties associated with measuring patient satisfaction, it is still viewed as a valuable undertaking by some. Having used patient satisfaction questionnaires to ascertain the needs of patients in an elderly unit, we felt that many patients were still reluctant to criticize the staff or environment, even though the questionnaire was sent to their home and was anonymous.

Our experience reinforces the findings of many others, in identifying that the expectations of many patients are low. We find that patients are often willing to excuse staff inefficiencies, possibly due to media information stating that the NHS is underfunded and the nursing and medical staff overworked. Many patients feel that staff are doing their best in stressful circumstances, but fail to mention even then how the service could be improved.

We feel that satisfaction questionnaires do play a part, but are limited in their ability to change and improve the quality of service offered to patients. Many patients often reiterate what staff have felt for a long time. There is a limit on the improvements that can be generated following such surveys if initiatives are not supported by Management who hold financial or other resources.

PEER REVIEW

Peer review is a situation where colleagues appraise each other's performance, or appraise a situation. It can take place by using a number of different techniques. These include interview situations, Slater rating scales and self-rating questionnaires.

The advantage of using peer review is that it is a method of evaluating an individual's performance which can encourage a nurse to consider professional accountability for his or her actions. However, in practice, when colleagues know each other well, it can be difficult for them to be constructive in giving criticism and any form of negative feedback without both individuals feeling that it is a personal slight. One might also feel that another colleague is subjective in views relating to a particular issue and thus the feedback would be of no benefit to the individual.

Having used peer review for colleague appraisal, we found the situation somewhat artificial. We found it difficult to be 'negative' about each other's work but also viewed our posts as learning experiences, and therefore will (to some degree) make mistakes. We felt that this method may be of use where people find self-appraisal difficult. We also found that the better you know a person socially, the more restricted your ability to criticize their work. It can be advantageous to use a colleague you respect, but who may not know you in a social capacity. This can be a more objective way of discussing one's work and inviting another colleague to comment upon situations without it being seen as criticism – it is simply another person's point of view.

COMPLAINTS PROCEDURE

The monitoring of complaints has been used by most hospitals in recent years as part of a QA strategy. In practice, this process can either be of extreme benefit to health authorities or of little value in the overall QA strategy. Sometimes one sees notices pinned on the walls of wards inviting both patients and visitors to write to the person in question with comments. Personally, we have found this way of encouraging complaints and comments of limited use. First, the print is usually too small and the posters often placed in unsuitable places. Second, the relatives are often loathe to criticize a ward when they see obvious problems of short staffing or lack of equipment and feel the staff are doing 'their best' within a certain situation.

However, one health authority decided to place boxes in lots of areas around the hospital, including the entrances, near the dining room, along the corridors, with large notices encouraging people to give their comments relating to the service of that hospital. This proved beneficial because the public had easy access to paper, pens and could then write comments as they passed.

Most areas have a complaints policy which is dealt with at a unit level. Our concern with complaints procedures is that the individual complaint may be dealt with, but the cycle of improvement does not necessarily begin following a complaint. For example, one gentleman complained that his elderly mother's false teeth had been mislaid in a transfer to another ward. The teeth could not be found and both wards blamed each other for the loss. The outcome was an apology from the unit, some new teeth for the elderly lady in question and a reminder to ward staff to take care of people's property. This situation could very well happen again because staff on both wards failed to identify:

- The policy for documenting patients' property.
- The policy for transferring patients between wards.
- The ward policy regarding safe storage of property.

These are 'process failures' due to lack of clear requirements. Two issues emerge from this incident: (i) the issues of account-ability, i.e. where an individual is responsible for following policies and procedures – this cannot occur in the absence of either of these documents; (ii) if incidents/accidents occur, and no change occurs to prevent them happening again, one has to question if staff really understand the use of a QA programme. Hence the above example cannot be classed as 'quality assurance' simply because of a quality assessment, as no improvements were instigated as a result.

CLINICAL INDICATORS

Having mentioned clinical indicators above, it is worth expanding on these and reviewing their use within a hospital context. A clinical indicator is defined as 'a measure of the clinical management and outcome of care'. Some of the measures will reflect outcome, for example, mortality and ward infection rates. Others may be process type indicators; an example could be the degree of compliance with criteria of admission to special units, or how long before medical staff assess a patient in the Accident and Emergency Department. The end product is the actual number of patients who fulfil or do not fulfil an indicator of care.

Utilization of expensive resources, such as unnecessary inves-tigations relating to X-ray, blood testing and urinalysis, can be identified, and are not only a misuse of resources but are not appropriate in terms of quality of care.

The requirements of a clinical indicator are:

- That information is available.
- That the indicator is relevant to the particular practice, e.g. it concerns a frequently treated condition or a major complica-tion.
- That the measure is achievable.

Clinical indicators should also be acceptable to health care providers as a reasonable measure of their performance. The

clinical indicators lies in the potential to provide an
ss to health care providers of their level of practice so
iere it is less than optimal, improvement will be facili-

Clinical indicators fall into two categories: 'rate-based' and
'sentinel event'. Rate-based indicators are those in which it is
common for a certain number of cases to be unfavourable. A
medical example would be a 5% infection rate for patients who
are post-operative from a cholycystectomy. The threshold for
infection may be 5%, and a percentage higher than this would
alert a department of potential problems. A nursing example
may be a 5% pressure sore incidence for a hospital, whereas a
10% indicates problems within certain areas of the hospital.

Sentinel events are those which happen rarely and which
describe a major event requiring individual investigation. A
medical example may be a maternal death, and a nursing
example may be a patient who dies as a result of receiving a
burn from stepping into a scalding hot bath.

Clinical indicators are useful for medical staff as they identify
possible problems where there are highly dependent patients or
high volume areas of patient care, thus reflecting the overall
standard of care. Trends may be explained by the severity of
the patient's illness or they may indicate a problem which
requires addressing.

Nurses may also find clinical indicators useful. However,
nursing is predominantly concerned with process and not
outcome criteria. As mentioned above, nurses cannot specify if
it is their intervention or the multidisciplinary team's intervention which has the most effect on patients. Nurses may need to
consider formulating clinical indicators on a multidisciplinary
basis. An example of this may be 'readmission rates due to poor
discharge planning'.

Nurses can identify many problems that are indicators of
poor clinical practice, and developing clinical indicators can
provide another method in improving the quality of care.

MEDICAL AUDIT IN THE NHS

Medical audit is 'the systematic, critical analysis of the quality
of medical care, including the procedures used for diagnosis

and treatment, the use of resources, and the resulting outcome and quality of life for the patient' (White paper, 1989).

Although according to some authors there have always been enthusiasts (Dalley, 1989) it was not until 1988 that the professional medical bodies became interested in audit, predominantly due to fear of external pressures from both the government (Shepherd, 1988) and the public (Griffiths, 1983). Some medical professionals were worried by external auditors and preferred the medical profession to be self-regulating rather than open to scrutiny by other professions (Gumpert, 1988).

A variety of methods of medical audit have been used in an attempt to meet the criteria as defined by the document *Working for Patients* (1989). The categories most common for audit tend to fall into the following four:

- Treatment – clinical, diagnostic.
- Communication – information to the patient and information concerning activity.
- Education – postgraduate.
- Financial – cost-effectiveness, e.g. guidelines for the use of investigations, policies on drugs, etc.

Published examples of audit include the number of deaths caused by asthma (Markowe, 1987) and the effectiveness of the discharge of elderly patients (Currie, 1984). The audit of perioperative deaths (Buck, 1987) is considered a valuable piece of work in changing practice but costs in excess of £200,000 to complete. In order for wide changing practice to occur from medical audit, more time and more effective information systems must be present within a hospital, as the current system of collating accurate data is slow, tedious and usually inaccurate.

Many medical staff are involved in medical audit, however, where this has failed to occur this may according to one author (Mckee, 1989), be due to any or all of the following reasons:

- A dislike of terms.
- A belief that quality is implicit within a medical professional's practice.
- Audit is time-consuming.
- The information currently available relates to activity rather than patient outcome.

- The areas that need change, e.g. better clerical support, lie outside a clinician's scope.

However, regardless of the above factors, medical staff are now beginning to share ideas and practice. An example of this is the Medical Audit Newsletter and the involvement of the Kings Fund in promoting and training medical staff in how to approach audit. As yet, there is little work published on medical staff working in a multidisciplinary audit setting nor of evaluation of interpersonal aspects of practice.

The use of quality initiatives, as mentioned above, can be of benefit but needs to be part of the organization's overall plan for quality assurance. Some authorities use specific frameworks to establish a structure whereby quality initiatives fit into the general framework and are not isolated incidents. The use of such frameworks will now be discussed.

FRAMEWORKS FOR QUALITY ASSURANCE

Approaches based on measurement cannot fully encapsulate the wide range of services offered in the NHS. There is a tendency to focus only on technical aspects of care, which are more easily measured, and this excludes interpersonal or expressive aspects of performance which have a major impact on the quality of care. Ginsberg and Hammans (1988) argue that an alternative to measurement, which is already in place, is providing health care givers with more and better information on the effectiveness of outcomes in medical procedures. Competitive approaches concentrate on outcome criteria, yet process criteria in the NHS (and particularly the nursing profession) are equally important elements.

A clear difference needs to be made between quality initiatives and a QA programme. Quality initiatives can be one-off events which arise in response to a problem or because staff feel an effort should be made to find out how effective their service is. Many nurses will introduce audit and standard-setting as an effort to demonstrate they are interested in reviewing their service. However, a QA programme is an approach for reviewing and improving the quality of service given. In order to develop a systematic approach, one can use established frameworks, such as Lang (1976) or Wilson (1987) or continue developing frameworks such as Maxwell (1984) and Donabedian (1966).

Maxwell (1984)

Maxwell (1984) recognized that, in a society where resources are limited, self-assessment by health care professionals is not satisfactory in demonstrating the efficiency or effectiveness of a service. Furthermore, quality of care cannot be measured by a single dimension such as the interpersonal aspects or the technical aspects. Maxwell proposed six other dimensions to quality, which need to be recognized and therefore require different assessment skills and, in turn, different measures. The dimensions of quality he proposed are:

- Access to service.
- Relevance to need (for the whole community).
- Effectiveness (for individual patients).
- Equity (fairness).
- Social acceptance.
- Efficiency and economy.

An example of applying these dimensions could be to an Outpatients' Department Service for Ear, Nose and Throat complications:

- *Access.* This could be determined by the time it took from visiting the General Practitioner to receiving an appointment to see a consultant.
- *Relevance to need.* Analysis of the size of the department for the community, the times it opened, the type and adequacy of equipment for specialist procedures would be undertaken.
- *Effectiveness.* This may be possibly determined by how many patients were treated successfully for a specific complaint.
- *Equity.* A method of assessing this may be to involve consumer groups and other professionals in research to find out if the service is 'fair' to all consumers.
- *Social acceptability.* This may relate to how the patient's dignity is protected whilst being examined, the availability of information leaflets in different languages, and issues such as disabled people having easy access to the department.

- *Efficiency and economy.* This may relate to the comparison of workload/cost with another ENT Unit of similar size.

Maxwell's point when suggesting the above dimensions is that in order to look at the quality of a service, one must examine how it performs as a whole, rather than at fragmented parts of it, such as how the staff communicate with patients, or one aspect, such as the interpersonal skills of the staff.

Wilson (1987)

Wilson's approach to quality assurance using the Adult Learning Method has been used extensively in Canada and is now currently in use in the UK. The model was formulated due to dissatisfaction with other QA models, which were laborious, demanding and required detailed documentation. The Adult Learning Model (ALM) is based on emphasis in management, standards being formulated and a good communication structure.

It is designed to be a strategy of growth based on communication and leadership, and the system is said to be capable of encompassing all mechanisms that are currently needed, such as audit and standard-setting (Harrison, 1988).

Wilson considers there to be four essential components to a departmental QA programme. These are:

- Setting objectives.
- Quality promotion.
- Activity monitoring.
- Performance assessment.

Wilson suggests that setting objectives comprises performance standards and management goals. A standard is described as 'a definition of attainment in the present', and should be written for immediate use. Quality promotion is prospective and relates to quality investment, activity monitoring concerns the control and supervision of quality and its concurrent and performance assessment is related to audit, and evaluation of activities.

Wilson's model begins with the writing of the department's mission statement and the listing of the principle functions, and what quality assurance/control monitoring is already in place. From here the department provides the QA committee with information from quality assessment procedures and develops a QA plan. The aim of the plan is to propose specific quality assurance procedures for all its principle functions. Following this, standards and criteria are developed for current assessment and a contract is drawn up, which is revised annually.

The principles of this model's success hinge on their approach to adults and how they learn. The approach introduces each level of the programme in a structured and reasonable way and is a modification of the old, and not an entirely new system. Top level support is essential and momentum is maintained by ensuring prompt feedback after each element of the plan is attained, and also to direct the next level of achievement. Adult learners, in Wilson's experience, are action-oriented and require an integration of their present skills and knowledge to a new theory. Thus, the strategy of this model is based on growth rather than the introduction of a new system.

Lang (1976)

An approach adopted by some authorities, and one that has appealed to the nursing profession, has been the framework for change formulated by Lang (1976). This framework has subsequently been adopted and developed by the American Nurses Association. The stages depicted in Figure 3.1 should be

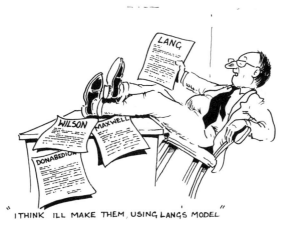

"I THINK ILL MAKE THEM, USING LANGS MODEL"

Illustration 3.2 Using Lang's model.

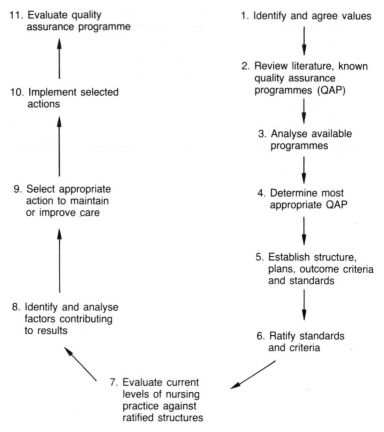

11. Evaluate quality assurance programme

1. Identify and agree values

10. Implement selected actions

2. Review literature, known quality assurance programmes (QAP)

3. Analyse available programmes

9. Select appropriate action to maintain or improve care

4. Determine most appropriate QAP

5. Establish structure, plans, outcome criteria and standards

8. Identify and analyse factors contributing to results

6. Ratify standards and criteria

7. Evaluate current levels of nursing practice against ratified structures

Figure 3.1 Lang's model for nursing quality assurance.

followed and, when the cycle is completed, the process should begin again.

Lang's (1976) framework can be used separately or in conjunction with the elements of 'structure, process and outcomes', which are the components of Donabedian's (1966) framework.

CRITIQUE OF FRAMEWORKS

The criteria below will be used to critique each of the above frameworks, as current literature suggests that the success of a QA programme depends upon the following:

- Economic and resource implications.
- The impact on organizational culture.
- The level of employee participation.
- The political environment.

Maxwell (1984)

Economic and resource implications

Maxwell's (1984) dimensions of health care quality can be applied (in theory) to any health care setting and at any level of the organization. His criteria can be applied from national to ward level situations in order to assess the quality of care.

If Maxwell's (1984) approach were to be applied at a regional level it would be a costly and time-consuming way of monitoring services and does not take into account the economic limitations health authorities face. Currently, access to services and relevance to need would be the most expensive dimensions to adjust and the least likely to be economically viable. However, in the long term, with more emphasis placed on efficient service planning and reviewing epidemiological changes, these dimensions could be fulfilled.

Impact on organizational culture

Maxwell's (1984) approach would suit many health care settings, although much more consideration of the consumer's point of view in terms of equity and social acceptability would need to be sought. This again would be a costly part of a QA programme, and the question of how one decides if the health care system passes or fails one of the dimensions remains unanswered. Maxwell (1984) does not put forward any ideas as to what would be the optimum standard in the dimensions of quality, nor does he state how they would be monitored.

Political environment

The framework could be applied regardless of the political influences of the time. However, it has been argued that the government focus in this political time rests heavily upon effi-

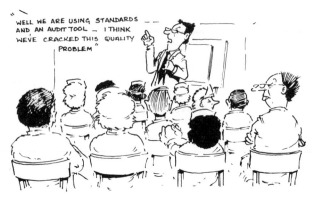

Illustration 3.3 Cracking the quality problem.

ciency and economy (Towell, 1988), and the other dimensions of quality such as social acceptability may be less important.

South East Staffordshire Health Authority used Maxwell's (1984) dimensions as an initial focus on their QA programme, and did so without any further resources. They later implemented a management development programme to support the quality initiatives.

Employee participation

Using Maxwell's model it is difficult to forecast the level of participation required by employees of the health authority. This approach would be difficult to implement at either ward or unit level due to fiscal restraints and lack of financial autonomy. This leads to the conclusion that Maxwell's theory could be useful in looking at planning health care services on a macro level, i.e. national and regional health care services, but not on a micro level, i.e. ward level.

Wilson (1987)

Economic and resource implications

Wilson's (1987) model could be one of the most useful methods for tackling problems within an organization, particularly when we consider that many *ad hoc* initiatives from most professional groups in the NHS are currently under way but not being viewed by senior management as to how they interrelate with each other.

This model potentially regulates initiatives and quality monitoring, as each department is responsible for developing the quality assurance plan with services. Therefore it is more likely to be reasonable, and within resource limitations.

Impact on the organizational culture

This model would obviously need senior management support in order to succeed. Whilst the development of standards, criteria, the QA plan and the review of the contract are feasible and achievable activities within the organization, the issue of change management following the identification of a problem after audit is not addressed. Protocols and procedures currently exist within the health service, although this is no guarantee that they will be followed. How 'change' occurs, and by whom, is one of the most important aspects of a QA programme and as such, Wilson's model (in failing to address this), may have limited organizational effects.

Level of employee participation

We recognize that, for any QA programme to be effective, senior management must be involved. The impact of this model on a hospital may leave many staff excluded from the development of standards and the QA plan. Heads of department are naturally going to be people such as the Ward Manager or the Senior Porter. However, many valuable activities are undertaken by ward nurses or radiographers or physiotherapists. The inclusion of all staff within some wards is not feasible using this model, due to the numbers of staff in some areas. However, that is not to dismiss its value in areas where participating with one's colleagues is more manageable, and there are fewer staff to give feedback following attending a QA session.

Political environment

This model of approaching quality assurance may not be affected by the changing political environment. The framework does not suggest concentrating on one process or dimension of quality but arises from the function of a department. Therefore, it is dependent on the key function and the goals to be achieved. If the goals change so will the functions and the subsequent QA plan.

Lang (1976)

Economic and resource implications

This is a comprehensive model, however; at a practical level it would be expensive to implement and, at a unit level, time-consuming before any results were achieved. If a hospital had many quality problems, the programme would take a great deal of time and effort to establish and maintain momentum.

Impact on the organizational culture

Although Lang's (1976) model has positive aspects (such as involving nurses and defining specific criteria to measure), it is limited, in that it does not encompass other aspects of the health service organization, such as access to service.

Level of employee participation

From a nursing perspective, Lang's model may have advantages as the level of involvement from staff could be high. Maintaining momentum may be difficult at ward level if problems take a long time to solve.

Political environment

Lang's model could be implemented regardless of political changes. It could also be transferable to various hospital settings.

Donabedian (1966)

Economic and resource implications

Using Donabedian's framework requires a great deal of time if the standards formulated are to be useful and of value. Organizations may find that this framework can be used not only as part of the QA programme but as a corporate approach in itself. Therefore, the framework has value. However, to use this method alone would not encompass all the measures required of a comprehensive quality assurance framework.

Impact on the organizational culture

Organizationally, although using this framework to write standards can be very positive, the standards need to interrelate with other developments to prevent duplication and the formulation of differing levels of standards.

Level of employee participation

All members of staff both nursing and from a multidisciplinary background can be involved in this framework of improving quality. Hospital members may recognize other factors such as 'structure' elements in how to improve care which they would not normally associate as relevant, particularly in nursing where the 'process' of care predominates.

Political environment

This method could be used regardless of the political environment; however, if resources are limited nurses may feel they have less control over structural elements, e.g. staffing levels, than they do over process elements. Furthermore, the underlying principles of setting 'achievable' standards in times of scarce resources are open to abuse.

Conclusion of critique

In conclusion to the above analysis of models, a model for the 1990s should:

- Be able to review all dimensions of services, as for example, in Maxwell's (1984) dimensions.
- Involve defining and measuring specific criteria outlined in Lang's (1976) model.
- Involve steps to continually monitor and improve quality.

- And be capable of adapting to political change and financial constraints.

However, none of the above models are sensitive enough to financial implications and resource difficulties. Nor do they look (with the exception of Maxwell's 1984 Model) specifically at the criteria that constitute a quality service from a patient/consumer perspective. A more comprehensive model could be a combination of the above, as well as further emphasis on outcomes of patient care.

ECLECTIC APPROACH FOR AN ORGANIZATION-WIDE QA PROGRAMME

Based on our practical experiences, this section aims to present a practical model that is flexible enough to use in a multi-disciplinary health care service. The interpretation of the model will depend on the political environment, the complexity of the organizational structure and other factors such as the size of the unit or the ward involved. This model aims to encourage a high level of employee and patient participation, and to be sensitive to fiscal restraints. This eclectic model would require management commitment and leadership with a strong emphasis placed on involvement and direction for all staff and patients. The model would be based on a system providing information on the quality of care and service and utilizing resources currently in place (Figure 3.2).

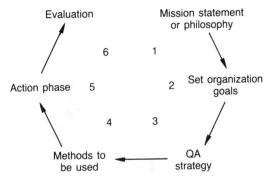

Figure 3.2 Stages of the quality assurance cycle.

Stage 1

One needs to identify the quality components in the hospital philosophy or mission statement. From our previous experience we have found this to be a useful and necessary undertaking, as very often patients' priorities and requirements are very different from employee requirements. Furthermore, organizational goals regarding the focus of quality need to be agreed and incorporated into the mission statement or hospital philosophy.

Stage 2

This involves setting objectives for QA that are closely aligned to the organizational goals. For example, there is little point in *ad hoc* groups carrying out 'sharing, caring' type QA initiatives for customer satisfaction if the organizational philosophy is based on seeing the highest possible number of patients. Therefore, in order to reduce waiting lists before a quality assurance strategy is formulated, the philosophy and objectives of the organization need to be understood and agreed. If these are not agreed initially, management and employees may lack commitment in meeting these objectives and the programme will have limited impact.

Stage 3

Senior staff within the organization should be involved in the development of a strategy for meeting objectives. This strategy should include the mission, the objectives and a long-term plan with time-scales. The role of the QA manager and the QA committee should be determined, so that there are clear lines of responsibility and accountability throughout the organization.

Stage 4

Tactics to be used in operationalizing the strategy need to be identified. These must include education of staff in the objectives and the tools and techniques of QA, communication, documentation and co-ordination of all other quality initiatives, such as peer review, quality circles, etc.

Stage 5

This is the action phase and implementation of the strategy.

Stage 6

Evaluate the QA programme and review the original organizational goals as well as the long-term plan.

Critique of the eclectic model

Economic and resource implications

As identified in Stage 2, this model needs to reflect the resources that are available within the organization in order to meet the organizational goals.

Impact on the organizational culture

Ensuring that senior staff are involved with the development of the quality assurance as well as staff at all levels of the organization has the potential to ensure a successful programme. Education of all staff offers potential to ensure the culture is receptive and proactive to the QA approach.

Political environment

The eclectic model should not be affected by the political environment, as the aims of the organization will determine how the QA strategy is developed and operationalized. The amount of resources will determine the scope of the tactics as outlined in Stage 4.

Employee participation

As well as encouraging and promoting a high degree of employee participation, the patients' views and priorities will be sought, as identified in Stage 1.

By agreeing initially the philosophy of the organization the quality assurance strategy will be congruent with the objectives recognized.

IS QUALITY ASSURANCE ENOUGH?

During this chapter we have given some examples of QA strategies and methods of how the concept of 'quality' can be attained.

What we find are numerous examples of initiatives that either form a total picture or are *ad hoc* in response to a crisis. However, although audit methods such as Monitor can help us remedy the 'process' element of care, they cannot always improve the 'expressive' component that is part of the service in the NHS. For example, many patients may have a dressing changed in the morning following analgesia to prevent discomfort. The nurse may use an aseptic technique, the appropriate wound dressing and carry out the procedure with efficiency. However, if that nurse fails to realize how the patient considers the impact of a wound on their self-esteem, or fails to show empathy and 'caring', the patient's view of their care as a whole can colour their whole experience of a hospital. Examples of trying to audit expressive elements such as 'Are nurses kind to patients?' are open to interpretation, e.g. in a rehabilitation setting the nurse may well try to be kind and want to test outcomes for that patient, but may be asking a patient to improve stamina by walking further distances. The patient may not see this as kindness, but as cruelty.

Thus, the essential personal qualities of staff must be present, and these cannot be necessarily controlled by an 'organization'. However, the philosophies that under-pin total quality management can, in fact, influence how staff are trained and what the emphasis of the organization is. If quality assurance is to become 'everybody's business,' a major rethink in the NHS has to take place, so much so that interpersonal aspects of care and service are to some degree controlled. For example, role modelling of key people such as ward sisters is of great importance. So too is the involvement of all staff in improving the service in situations such as quality circles. Therefore, support from the top, clear leadership, training of all staff, and an awareness of what 'quality' is, based on the views of customers, is the beginning of determining the standards that need to be set for and delivered to customers of the NHS. This cannot be achieved by *ad hoc* initiatives or by one person in an organization trying to do this. It can only be achieved by the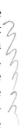

organization, i.e. the whole hospital, adopting a comprehensive approach.

CONCLUSION

Critics such as Sarsfield (1973) have argued that QA frameworks have not managed to assign a sufficiently prominent role to the patient; nor have they been able to demonstrate how patient encounters relate to the health care system as a whole. Waters (1986) stresses that in using frameworks there are deficiencies in nursing knowledge in terms of providing data on expected outcomes, and also the tendency for nurses to set unrealistic goals for patient recovery.

QA programmes alone are not the answer for long-lasting hospital-wide quality improvement. The reasons for this are that, in our experience, *ad hoc* initiatives may work well in one area for a short period of time but often the same problems occurred repeatedly and clinical practice does not always improve after auditing. Other factors, such as planning and managing change following problem identification, were important and vital for the success of a QA programme. This will now be discussed in Chapter 4.

REFERENCES

Abdellah, F.G. (1958) *Effects of Nursing Staffing on Satisfaction with Nursing Care.* Monograph. American Hospitals Association.

Abdellah, F.G. and Levine, G. (1957) What patients say about their nursing care. *Hospitals, JAHA,* **31**, 41–8.

Benner, P. (1984) *From Novice to Expert – Excellence and Power in Clinical Practice.* Addison Wesley, New York.

Buck, N. (1987) *Report of a Confidential Enquiry into Perioperative Deaths.* Nuffield Provincial Hospitals, Kings Fund, London.

Caddow, P. (1986) 'Questions on quality'. *Nursing Times,* **September 10**, 44–8.

Carr-Hill, R. (1989) Too simple for words. *Health Service Journal.* **June 15th**

Cartwright, A. (1964) *Human Relationships and Hospital Care.* Routledge, Kegan and Paul, London.

Crosby, P. (1979) *Quality is Free.* Heinmann Publishing, London.

Crown, J. (1989) Proof of the pudding. *Health Service Journal,* **99**(5166), 1070–1.

Currie, C.T. (1984) Elderly patients discharged from an accident and emergency department – their dependency and support. *Archives of Emergency Medicine,* **1**, 205–13.

Dalley, G. (1989) *Quality Management Initiatives*. Draft Survey Report, Centre for Health Economics, York University, York.

Davies, C. (1985) *Can Quality Circles add to the Quality of Life in the Health Service*. Kings Fund Centre (conference paper), London.

Department of Health (1992) *Patients' Charter* HMSO, London.

Donabedian, A. (1966) Evaluating the quality of medical care. *Millbank Memorial Fund Quarterly*, **44** (part 2) 166–206.

Ginsberg, B. and Hammans, G. (1988) Competition and the quality of care – the importance of information. *Inquiry*, **Spring**, 108–115.

Glennester, H. (1986) *The Nursing Management Function After Griffiths. A Study in N.W. Thames* (interim report). North West Thames Health Authority.

Griffiths, R. (1983) *NHS Management Inquiry*. DHSS circular, HMSO, London.

Gumpert, J. (1988) Why on Earth do Surgeons Need Quality Assurance? *Royal College of Surgeons*, **70**, 85–92.

Harrison, A. (1988) An approach to a quality assurance programme. *NAQA Journal Conference Proceedings*, **November**, 22.

Hyde, P. (1984) Quality circles, one – something for everyone. *Nursing Times*, **November 28**, 49–51.

Incomes Data Services Ltd (1985) *Study 352: Quality Circles*. Incomes Data Services Ltd, London.

Johnson, D. (1984) Quality circles three – a team approach to care. *Nursing Times*, **December 5**, 36–8.

Johnson, D. and Clarke, V. (1984) Quality circles, two – developing quality of care. *Nursing Times*, **December 5**, 36–8.

Kitson, A. (1986) Methods of measuring quality. *Nursing Times*, **August 27**.

Lang, N.M. (1976) Quality Assurance – the Idea and its Development in the United States, in *Measuring the Quality of Care* (eds M. Willis and M. Linwood), Churchill Livingstone, Edinburgh.

McGhee, A. (1961) *The Patient's Attitude to Patient Care*. E and S Livingstone, Edinburgh.

McKee, C. (1989) Medical audit – a review. *Journal of the Royal Society of Medicine*, **82**, 475–9.

Markowe, H. (1987) Controlled investigation of deaths from asthma in hospitals in the North East Thames Region. *British Medical Journal*, **294**, 1255–8.

Maxwell, R.J. (1984) Quality assessment in health. *British Medical Journal*, **12 May**, 1470–2.

Moores, B. and Thompson, A. (1985) What 1357 hospitals think about aspects of stay in British acute hospitals. *Journal of Advanced Nursing*, **11**, 87–102.

Moore, J. (1988) *Quality of Service – Patients as People*. Speech to the Office of Health Economics, 5th July.

Nehring, V. and Geach, B. (1973) Patients' education of their care and why they don't complain. *Nursing Outlook*, **21**(5), 317–21.

Pursig, R. (1974) *Zen and the Art of Motorcycle Maintenance*. Vintage Publications, London.

Raphael, W. (1967) *Patients and Their Hospitals – A Survey of Patients' Views of Life in General Hospitals.* King Edward Hospital Fund for London, London.

RCN (1980) Standards of Care. Royal College of Nursing, London.

RCN (1981) *Towards standards.* Royal College of Nursing, London.

Reid, E. (1986) Performance indicators. *Nursing Times,* **10 September,** 44–8.

Sale, D. (1988) Down Dorset way. *Nursing Times,* **84**(28), 31–3.

Salmon, (1966) *Report on Senior Nurse Staffing Structure.* HMSO, London.

Sarsfield, C. (1973) Health service research – a working model. *New England Journal of Medicine,* **289,** 132.

Shepherd, G. (1988) Information please. *Times Health Supplement,* **5**(2), 7.

Towell, D. (1988) *An Ordinary Life in Practice – Developing Comprehensive Community Based Services for Older People with Learning Disabilities.* Kings Fund, London.

Value for Money (1991) HMSO, London.

Ventura, M.R. (1982) A Patient Satisfaction Measure as a Criteria to Evaluate Primary Nursing. *Nursing Research,* **31**(4), 226–30.

Vetter, N. (1986) Performance indicators in care of the elderly. *Nursing Times,* **1 April,** 30–2.

Virtue of Patients (1991) *Making Best Use of Nursing Resources.* HMSO, London.

Waters, K. (1986) Cause and Effect. *Nursing Times,* **January 29,** 28.

White Paper (1989) *Working for Patients.* HMSO, London.

Williamson, J.W. (1988) *Improving Medical Practice and Health Care.* Ballinger Publishing Company, Cambridge, MA.

Wilson, C. (1987) *Hospital-wide Quality Assurance: Models for Implementation and Development.* W.B. Saunders, Toronto.

WHO (1985) *WHO Euro Reports – The Principles of Quality Assurance.* Regional Office for Europe, Copenhagen.

Wysenewski, L. (1988) The Emphasis on Measurement in Quality Assurance. Reasons and Implications. *Inquiry 25,* **Winter,** 424–36.

4

Managing change

Previous chapters have identified a variety of approaches aimed at improving the quality of care patients receive in hospital. Inherent in all such initiatives is the assumption that there is always room for improvement. Many nurses, in recognition of this assumption, have been exploring different systems of delivering care to patients, in the belief that some of these offer the opportunity to improve the quality of nursing care patients receive. Whether setting standards, auditing, devising a quality assurance strategy or changing the system of care delivery, new goals and levels of attainment will need to be set and monitored. Meeting these goals requires changes to be made. Managing change can be a difficult and painful process, and the success or failure of initiatives such as these will depend on how well that change is instigated.

In our experience, changing the system of care delivery on a ward to one of primary nursing proved to be one of the most challenging innovations we have attempted to manage in our careers. This chapter, and chapter 5, therefore explore the process of managing change, using our practical experience of implementing Primary Nursing into the clinical area. We refer to this process as changing the work methodology. This is because it may not always be possible (for reasons identified later) to reach the goal of primary nursing but, nevertheless, significant quality improvements can be achieved in the attempt.

In order to instigate these changes it is useful to have some knowledge of some of the theories of change outlined in the literature. The first section therefore gives a brief resumé of some of these theories. No critique of these is presented, as it was not intended to debate the finer academic points of one theory versus another. Instead, we explain how we have integrated some of the theories we have found useful into our framework for changing the work methodology on the ward.

DEFINING 'CHANGE'

In searching for a definition of 'change' Gillies (1989) notes that it is both a noun and a verb. The noun refers to an alteration; the verb refers to the process of alteration. 'Change' is therefore defined as 'the process of moving from one system to another.' This definition is useful, as it requires the change agent to consider input, throughput, output and feedback loops of both the present system and that which the manager hopes will exist in the future.

The phenomenon of change has been explored using a variety of theoretical models, including the sociological, psychological and organizational or systems perspective. Imershein (1977) deductively utilizing the work of Kuhn, conceptualized the process of change in scientific and technological areas in terms of a paradigm shift. Innovation occurs in a fairly revolutionary form when the existing paradigm is no longer able to provide answers for significant problems. Imershein acknowledges an in-built resistance to change, suggesting, as an immediate response, that minor alterations are attempted within the existing paradigm in an attempt to solve recalcitrant problems. When these fail, there will be a search for a new paradigm to accommodate both the already manageable, and the now unmanageable problems. This leads to a revolutionary shift to the new paradigm. Within this context, major innovations therefore tend to occur against a background of crisis, at a time when tensions are often high.

Sociologists define three basic stages of change: (i) initiation, which involves the launching of new ideas; (ii) legitimatation, which involves the arguments for change being communicated; and (iii) congruence, the process of reconciling the value systems of those proposing the change with those who are the targets of the change.

These stages have been utilized by Cuba and Clark (1978) in their procedural taxonomy for effecting change; namely: research, development, dissemination, demonstration, implementation, and institutionalization.

Another perspective on the change process is offered by the

systems theory. This is derived from social science, and contends that society is a series of interdependent units and systems, whose very existence depends on the nature of various sociable relationships.

The usefulness of this theory lies in its ability to show that everything is related in some way to something else. Systems theory explains social change through its conceptualization of an equilibrium. According to Homans (1981):

> The state of elements that enter the system and the mutual relationships between them is such that any change in one of the elements will be followed by changes in the other elements, tending to reduce the amount of that change.

In the exploratory stages of our move towards Primary Nursing, we became aware that it could not be viewed as an isolated initiative that would impact only the trained nurses on one ward. We were influenced significantly by the systems theory, which underpinned the assessment tool we developed to identify, plan and evaluate the factors that we saw as instrumental in moving us towards Primary Nursing.

We then examined theories that could help us to identify the variables that could influence the change process. Any change strategy is directed at changing human behaviour. As Plant (1987, p.21) observed, 'Unless behaviour changes, nothing changes'. The change process within an organization is therefore affected by the individuals within it. This is explored by Dyer (1984, p.4), who reflected that the organization is:

> . . . an abstraction. Organizations do not change their behaviour, although change in organizational structure or process can impact behaviour. What actually occurs is that a collection of people who share common orientations consciously or unconsciously decided . . . to change.

This observation was borne out by our own experiences in changing clinical practice at ward level. Knowledge of how we could create the environment where the individuals in the team felt motivated to take the decision to change was an essential element in helping us devise a strategy for change.

Basset (1971) offered insight into how this could be achieved. At the individual level, three elements are identified as prerequisites in order for change to occur. These are:

- The rational element (the recognition that change must occur).
- The affective element (the acceptance of the need for change at an emotional level).
- The achievement element (the belief that effective change is possible and the individual can contribute to it).

Other authors have made similar observations. Dalton (1970) identified that, for the change agent to take action, the individual had to perceive 'a felt need' strong enough to motivate him or her. This notion underpins most of the popular theories on models of management behaviour, which all have a disparity condition built into them. They are based on the assumption that the change strategy will involve the individual seeing the difference between what they are doing and what they should, or could, be doing. Management development programmes often involve an examination of the minimum/maximum positions of that particular theory with the aim of pushing the individual to the upper end of the continuum (Table 4.1).

Table 4.1 Maximum and minimum positions in McGregor's management theory (adapted from Dyer, 1984)

Theorist	Minimum position	Maximum position
Douglas McGregor	*Theory X* Assumption that managers had about people–they dislike work, want security, need direction and want direction	*Theory Y* Asumption of managers–the worker likes work, is self-motivated and accepts responsibility

Rogers (1979) expands these stages and identifies five phases through which the individual has to move (Figure 4.1). Rogers' theory is underpinned by two factors. First, the individual needs to be interested in the innovation, and second, they need to be committed to making the change occur.

It was apparent to us that if we were to instigate the change to Primary Nursing with the co-operation of staff, we had to ensure that our change plan gave consideration to overcoming

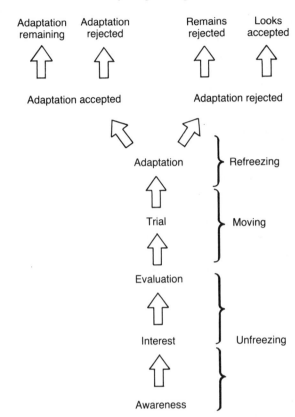

Figure 4.1 Roger's theory of change (from Welch, 1979).

the potential problems of staff who had not internalized the need for change by passing through the stages mentioned by the above theorists. We have therefore included strategies for helping staff to make this transition by moving them through these stages. These strategies were designed with the knowledge that individuals respond differently to change.

Pratt (1982) defines five categories into which individuals may fall, based on their response to the change process within the organization. These are:

- Enthusiasts – the initiators of the change. These may hold subordinate positions within the organization.
- Supporters – who are often respected and powerful members of the organization. Their views may be less radical than the

former group, but they are easily persuaded with the arguments for the need to change.

- Acquescers – who tend to follow the line of least resistance and adopt the change, even if only superficially, in response to pressure from the supporters.
- Laggards – who tend to be introspective and are unable to take a global view of the need for change. They tend to be sceptical and reject change until it is widely accepted by their peers.
- Antagonists – who actively or passively resist all change attempts as they are introduced.

Using this theory, it was clear that a number of differing tactics to instigate the change to Primary Nursing were required to embrace the needs of all the staff, assuming a wide range of responses to change based on Pratt's categories. However, from our experience of managing teams working in a clinical setting, we were aware of the limitations of devising a strategy based purely on individual responses. Other variables also needed to be considered.

The first such variable was the influence the team has on the attitudes and behaviour of the individual. Hawthorne (in Dyer, 1984) demonstrated that individuals can be, and often are, influenced in their judgments, decisions and actions by the way group members behave towards them. It may not be possible to predict the changes to specific individuals, but an overall effect can be seen.

Fretwell's (1985) demographic model of change (Figure 4.2) offers insight into factors that can move teams through the change process.

Key factors from this model that we identified as crucial for the successful implementation of Primary Nursing were:

- Consultation.
- Support.
- Praise.
- Peer groups.
- Teamwork.
- Anxiety controlled.

Having considered the influence that individuals and group responses might have on ensuring the success or failure of our

DEMOGRAPHIC MODEL OF CHANGE

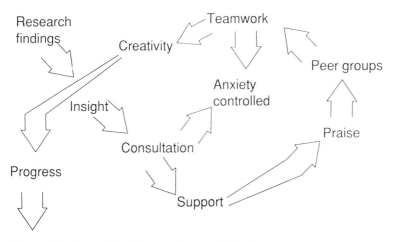

Figure 4.2 Fretwell's demographic model of change (from Fretwell, 1985).

change to Primary Nursing, we explored other variables that may affect our aim.

Stocking (1984), in her studies of innovation within the NHS, reiterated some of the themes of earlier theories, but introduced some other factors for consideration. She identified that, to make an innovation diffuse, some or all of the following would have to be evident:

- Identifiable enthusiasts – individuals who invented or discovered the idea, who are keen to disseminate it, and who put in considerable time and energy promoting it.
- Lack of conflict – with current national policies or established climates of opinion among professionals and other groupings.
- Local appeal – the innovation should appeal to those who have the power to promote change.
- Relevance – the innovation should meet the perceived needs of patients and staff. It should not require major role or attitude changes and should be simple to organize.
- Adaptability – the innovation should suit local circumstances.

- Little finance or other resource should be required – unless such requirements can be hidden or increase resources made available.

At a local level, this raised some interesting issues, which it became apparent that our change management plan would need to address.

First, although there was a body of opinion growing in the nursing profession that Primary Nursing was a worthwhile aim, there was by no means a consensus. Other professionals working as part of our multidisciplinary team also had reservations about the transition to the new method of working. Part of our strategy, therefore, had to include actions for influencing the climate of opinion amongst these groups.

Second, we needed to address the issue (identified by Stocking) of Primary Nursing having local appeal to those with the power to promote change. This was closely linked with her final identified factor – the availability of finance and resources. We were aware that there was a need for finance and resources that were necessary to make the change to Primary Nursing. To secure these, it was essential to gain support from those with the power to allocate them.

One model that particularly appealed to us when we were attempting to design a framework for identifying factors for consideration when changing to Primary Nursing was Lewins' (1953) forcefield analysis. This provides a framework for planned change and problem solving.

As shown in Illustration 4.1, the status quo is maintained when restraining forces equal the driving forces, and change will only occur when this balance is altered. When planning change, the change agents need to identify the driving and restraining forces, and to assess their relative strengths. These can be ranked in order of significance to restraining or driving the change.

These concepts were extremely important in helping us to plan strategies to reduce the restraining forces, and strengthen the driving forces that could assist us to reach our 'desired level'.

Lewin identified three stages of the change process: (i) unfreezing: (ii) moving to a new level; and (iii) refreezing.

The first – unfreezing – involves the process of becoming

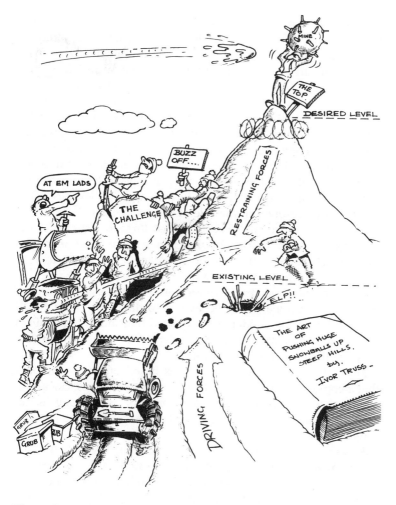

Illustration 4.1 Lewin's forcefield analysis.

aware of the problem and the need for change. There is also a need to believe that there is potential for improvement before the change process can progress. 'Moving to a new level' involves clarifying the problem and planning action, which involve 'identification' and 'scanning'. Identification involves subjects being influenced by someone who has power, or for whom they have respect. Scanning involves seeking information about potential options from a variety of sources (Marriner

Tomey, 1988, p.283). We saw identification and scanning as offering potential for influencing our staff when considering the change to Primary Nursing. A variety of strategies were found to be useful in providing staff with information in this opinion forming stage. 'Refreezing' is the integration of the change into one's personality and the constant stabilization of the change.

The final variable we identified as offering the potential to impact on our process of changing to Primary Nursing was the role of the change agent (ourselves). It was clear to us that we needed to develop skills and identify approaches that would help us to achieve the desired change. The following theories and approaches were influential in helping us to identify action required by ourselves in the role of the change agent.

Chin (in Bennis et al., 1988) identified three key strategies that can be used as approaches by the change agent when managing change. These are: (i) empirical rational; (ii) normative re-educative; and (iii) power coercive.

Empirical rational strategies are based on the assumption that people are rational and behave according to rational self-interest. Using this model, it is expected that individuals will be willing to adopt change if they accept that it is justified, and they see they will benefit from it.

Normative re-educative strategy is based on the assumption that people act according to their commitment to sociocultural norms. The rationality and intelligence of individuals is not entirely excluded, but attitudes and values are also taken into consideration.

Power coercive strategy involves compliance by the less powerful to the leadership of the more powerful. Conflict is a common feature of this strategy. The conflict theory of social change contends that at the basis of most organizational change is some form of conflict, i.e. dissatisfaction, alienation and frustration experienced by members of the organization. These members, in order to resolve or eliminate these conflicts attempt to change the circumstances within the organization. These efforts of change will usually lead to conflict with other groups who do not perceive any difficulties with the existing system.

We identified strategies for change using both the empirical rational, and normative re-educative approach.

Another strategy advocated by many authors is the notion of 'ownership' of the change by the individuals it will affect. This stems from early studies by Coch and French (1948), who identified the importance of involving everyone to be affected in the change plan. In this industrial-based research, methods that used little or no worker participation led to worker resistance, turnover and production loss; the trial group showed the fastest rate of relearning and surpassed previous output by 14% in 30 days. There were no resignations, no absenteeism and no grievances in the trial group. Plant (1987, p.23) emphasizes the importance of worker involvement as crucial to the likelihood of long-term behaviour change by showing it at points along a continuum (Figure 4.3). Gillies, (1989) extends this further by incorporating a feedback loop into the process.

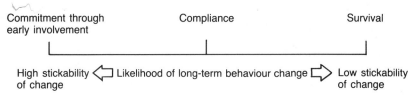

Figure 4.3 The change continuum (from Plant, 1987).

A change strategy that incorporates this philosophy of 'ownership' is the change agent model, which focuses on the use of communication skills and the development of a good working relationship between the leader (or change agent) and the person or people of the target system. Drawing on a normative, re-educative strategy, five steps are described (Tappen, 1989):

- Step 1 – build a relationship. This cites the need to build trust and respect. Actions recommended to achieve this include good communication techniques, openness, honesty, providing information on your skills and credentials and demonstration of ability.
- Step 2 – diagnose the problem. This is the identification of the 'felt need' to change. Methods used include meetings, conferences, informal discussions, surveys and questionnaires. Consensus building is also stressed.
- Step 3 – Assess resources. This includes motivation and commitment to change, knowledge and skills needed to implement the actual change behaviour, sources of power and

influence that support the change, economic resources available, time and energy available and social roles, norms and values that support the change.

- Step 4 – set goals and select strategies.
- Step 5 – stabilize, consolidate and reinforce the change.

The strategies we used for implementation of Primary Nursing were dominated by actions designed to fulfil the key factors identified as important by the above theorists, namely staff 'ownership' of the change, establishing and maintaining a helping relationship with those affected by the change and the use of a systematic approach to assessing, planning, implementing and evaluating the change.

APPLYING THE THEORY IN PRACTICE

Our initial drive to examine the change theories was a direct response to our previous attempts at change. Our early kamikaze-like 'missions' (as we came to regard them) of change tended to be launched with the accuracy of a Scud missile. We weren't really sure of our aim, we'd no way of knowing when we'd hit the target and, to make matters worse, we didn't seem to know who our allies were as they all wore the same uniforms. Furthermore, just when we were winning the battle, someone else would come and give us a new target and change half the troops!

Looking at Lewin's model (Illustration 4.1), at first, it is easy to dismiss it as almost too simplistic. On reflection, we realized this was its strength and our weakness. It is painfully obvious that, for every potential change, there are going to be things that will make it succeed (Lewin's 'driving forces') and things that make it fail (the 'restraining forces'). Although aware of this, we had not really analysed these. To return to the earlier analogy, this meant we were continually stumbling across hidden landmines, and missed out on the help of potential allies.

We also realized that in order to alter the work methodology on the ward, there were a huge number of other things within the management of the ward that would have to change to accommodate the new approach. These ranged from things as basic as what beds to use for which primary nurse's patients to more complex issues such as nurse accountability. This led to us referring back to the literature on the systems theory. We began to appreciate that there were a number of factors that could have a profound influence on the development of the new work methodology.

Similarly, the new work methodology could have far-reaching implications in altering a number of elements of the ward routine and other factors that we had not considered previously. The change process was therefore not just a simple exercise that affected a few trained nurses who wanted to introduce primary nursing. It involved a complex series of interrelationships between a number of factors. For every single one of these, there would be 'driving' and 'restraining' forces. If our goal was to be reached, we would have to identify all of these, and manage them effectively.

We likened some of our early efforts at managing the transition to primary nursing to sitting out in the sun. It was a hot and sticky business, and you never knew that you'd overdone it until you got burnt. In our efforts to protect ourselves against the unpleasant effects of an overdose of change, we identified a number of 'factors' that could offer us protection if applied into the process of changing the work methodology (Graham, 1991). In our experience it helps to consider these factors along with respective driving and restraining forces prior to implementing the new work methodology.

- Factor 1   Change management theory.
- Factor 2   Work methodology.
- Factor 3   Nursing role.
- Factor 4   Nurse accountability.
- Factor 5   Environment.
- Factor 6   Workload systems.
- Factor 7   Leadership style.
- Factor 8   Communications.
- Factor 9   Quality assurance.

This list is by no means exhaustive, but these are factors we ignored at our own expense. The purpose of exploring these factors is not to provide all the answers, or the 'right way' to manage the change. These will vary according to the culture of the ward concerned. The purpose is to help others to ask the right questions prior to changing the work methodology in their area.

One of the early difficulties we experienced was the lack of some kind of concrete focus from which we could work. Having read the theories on primary nursing, we needed a starting point, something we could refer to, channel our energies and start some action.

We developed the assessment tool shown in Table 4.2 to provide such a focus. Into this assessment tool we incorporated a concept we found useful from the literature review on change theory – that of the change continuum (Figure 4.3; Plant, 1987). This model reflected our own early experiences with quality assurance tools, namely, if staff are involved and consulted, any resultant changes they made as a result tended (in Plant's words) to 'stick.' However, the '4F's' hit squad style of quality assurance (find 'em, frighten 'em, freaten 'em and forget 'em), tended to have little long-lasting positive changes on clinical practice as a result.

In our assessment tool, for each of the factors, there are two possible extremes along a continuum. For example, for 'leadership style', at one end of the continuum there is an autocratic approach, at the other, a democratic approach. Having identified the two extremes, the change agent can identify, first, roughly whereabouts on the scale the current leadership style on the ward falls, and second, whereabouts on the scale the style needs to be if primary nursing is to be introduced. This can be completed for each of the factors. We find this tool useful in identifying how much work needs to be done in moving each factor to its ideal place on the scale.

It is also useful in the team building stage, where the team can identify the driving and restraining forces involved in changing each particular factor. Strategies can then be devised to maximize the driving forces and minimize the restraining forces. Obviously, such a scoring system is bound to be subjective, and this tool was not designed to become a scientific instrument. It is designed to serve as a focus for discussion on the nine factors, from which an implementation plan can be drawn up.

The next section therefore explores each of these factors (with the exception of quality assurance, which was covered in Chapter 3), looking at why they are important when considering changing the work methodology on the ward, and the practical approaches we found helped to move the different

Table 4.2 Nine-factor assessment tool for preparing from Primary Nursing

	Minimum position	Rating scale	Maximum position
Change management theory	Power coercive Theory X	-5 -4 -3 -2 -1 0 1 2 3 4 5	Normative Re-educative Theory Y
Work methodology	Task Allocation Work routine and task centred	-5 -4 -3 -2 -1 0 1 2 3 4 5	Primary nursing Work dynamic and patient centred
Nursing role	Role restricted Emphasis on technical skills	-5 -4 -3 -2 -1 0 1 2 3 4 5	Role expanded Nursing an intellectual activity Emphasis on creativity
Accountability	Diffuse Defence to medicine	-5 -4 -3 -2 -1 0 1 2 3 4 5	Nurse accountable Nurse autonomous
Leadership style	Autocratic	-5 -4 -3 -2 -1 0 1 2 3 4 5	Democratic
Workload systems	'Top Down' implementation and control	-5 -4 -3 -2 -1 0 1 2 3 4 5	'Bottom Up' implementation Owned by staff
Environment	Little devolution of responsibility Limited control	-5 -4 -3 -2 -1 0 1 2 3 4 5	Staff empowered to influence environment
Communications	Passive information Poor channels of organizational communication Poor interpersonal skills	-5 -4 -3 -2 -1 0 1 2 3 4 5	'Active' information Good channels of organizational communication Well developed interpersonal skills
Quality assurance	Initiative led	-5 -4 -3 -2 -1 0 1 2 3 4 5	Culture led/Total Quality Management

factors from left to right along the continuum on the assessment tool.

FACTOR 2: WORK METHODOLOGY

For all nurses involved in caring for patients, there is a need to organize that care in an appropriate and logical way. The work by Benner (1984), outlined in her book *From Novice to Expert* illustrates how, as the nurse becomes more expert, much of this organization becomes instinctive and intuitive. Hence dressings are taken off before Doctor's rounds, and redressed afterwards, analgesia is given prior to painful procedures and so on. Similarly, there is a need to organize the management of the ward, and the allocation of duties needed to enable the ward to function safely, effectively, and within a set budget, in an appropriate and logical way.

Throughout our student years, we experienced a wide variety of clinical placements, on some of which getting through a shift without going into the sluice for regular periods of unobserved hysteria was considered a major achievement. Yet on other wards, things seemed to run much more smoothly, and were 'nicer' places to work. At first, one tended to fall in with the masses and blame lack of staff for the former scenario. What became apparent to us as we became more experienced was that it was not always the best staffed wards that ran like clockwork. We also noticed a difference in the sort of work we were doing.

On some wards, there was a huge book with yellowed, curling pages around which all the nurses would cluster at the beginning of a shift. From this font of knowledge, our daily tasks would be assigned. Once completed, we would tick them in the book with a red pen especially assigned for the purpose. Evidence of a day's work depended on a neat row of red ticks.

Such an approach had its advantages. First, it meant you didn't need to think about what you had to do. This was very reassuring on a new ward, where the 'routine' was as yet unknown and a lot of time could be spent worrying about what we should be doing. Second, it meant all the work in the book was done. This would be a big advantage to the patients and the Ward Sister, whilst we functioned in a prenovice stage, still reeling from a 6-week introductory block of dictated notes on anatomy and physiology, and about as much intuition as a lemon.

On other wards, we were given certain patients to 'see to'. Sometimes we worked with a trained nurse, which was an advantage, as they would tell us what needed 'seeing to'. Although more challenging, this approach enabled us to build-up a good rapport with 'our' patients. This seemed to increase our job satisfaction but, at times, also our stress levels.

What was common on all of these wards, was that the work was assigned in pretty much the same way, regardless of who was on duty. Carrying on with the 'ward routine' became an accepted part of our early careers. It was not until we reached Sister level, and were given responsibility for organizing the methods to ensure patients received the best possible standard of nursing care, that we actually appreciated the importance of examining different methods of care delivery. At the same time we were also faced with equally important issues, such as developing staff, improving relationships with other members of the multidisciplinary team, and, in one area in particular, improving the standard of information given to patients (Evans and Hind, 1985). Referring back to the theories of change, we were perhaps searching for our new paradigm against a background of crisis (Imershein, 1977). The introduction of the nursing process, and the concept of individualized patient care; coupled with the declarations that all nursing care should be research based, meant that the task allocation system was at odds with these new ideas. It seemed to us that another method of organizing work needed to be found.

We embarked on a fact-finding exercise on differing methods of care delivery. We distilled all this new knowledge, and concluded (very crudely) that we actually had a choice of three methods:

- *Task allocation*. This, we found, was the official term given to our early experiences with the daily work book. It is the practice of allocating nursing work on the basis of the work to be performed. For example, doing 'rounds', such as the 'back' round, the drug round, the 'obs' round, etc. Such an approach has a number of advantages and disadvantages, some of which are noted below (Macdonald 1988).
  (i) Advantages (Goodman, in Macdonald, 1988)

- Staff soon gain competence in a particular task.
- It is an effective method of delegating work to staff with less training who may not identify the task needs doing.
- Everyone knows who is responsible for which task.

(ii) Disadvantages (Manthey, 1980)
- The focus of the work becomes the task, rather than the patient as a whole.
- This fragmentation of care may mean that no integrated picture of the patient's physical and psychological state is acquired.
- It can be monotonous for the nurse, and does not encourage application of nursing knowledge.

- *Team nursing/patient allocation.* Team nursing is the practice of allocating nursing work to a group of nurses who share the care of patients between the team on a patient allocated basis. The literature tends to refer to more formal teams, with clear delineation of small groups of nurses. In our experience, a less formal approach is common in many adult wards in general hospitals in the UK. Typically, two or three staff may be assigned to a particular bay or side of a ward, usually relating to the geographical layout. The composition of the teams changes frequently, as do the patients cared for by certain teams (Hegyvary and Goodman, in Macdonald, 1988):

(i) Advantages
- It enables nurses to care for the 'whole' patient, and integrate the knowledge gained into a comprehensive plan of care.
- It promotes continuity of care if nurses are allocated the same patients on a regular basis.
- It allows sharing of knowledge and expertise between staff.
- It facilitates the supervision of nursing aides and students.

(ii) Disadvantages
- It relies on the expertise of the team leader to plan and organize care. This can prove problematic on wards with only one trained nurse per shift.
- It can quickly disintegrate into task allocation, i.e. one

nurse in the team helps all the patients to wash, whilst the other does all the dressings or observations.
- Practised in its 'pure' sense it can make off-duty planning difficult.
- *Primary Nursing*. There has been a wealth of literature on this method in recent years. It has been described as 'The delivery of comprehensive, co-ordinated, continuous and individualized total patient care through the professional nurse who has autonomy, accountability and authority on a 24 hour basis' (Manthey, 1980).

Advantages and disadvantages are currently being hotly contested, some (cited in Macdonald, 1988) are:

(i) Advantages
- It increases job satisfaction for nursing staff (Steckel et al.; Fairbanks, in Macdonald, 1988).
- It improves patient satisfaction (Daeffler, in Macdonald, 1988; Giovennetti, 1986).
- It improves the standard of nursing care (Sellick et al.; Daeffler, in Macdonald, 1988).
- It increases the professional status of the nursing profession (Hegyvary in Macdonald, 1988; Manthey, 1980).

(ii) Disadvantages
- It is more stressful for nursing staff (Hegyvary, in Macdonald, 1988).
- It relies on a predominance of Registered General Nurses, which may make it more expensive (Giovennetti, 1986).
- There is as yet only a limited amount of research into benefits of this method.

This last criticism raises some interesting debates as to whether Primary Nursing should be widely adopted. Interestingly, in spite of an extensive literature search, there appears to be no more research on the impact of task allocation or the hybrid forms of patient allocation and team nursing. From a research-based perspective it is very much a case of swapping the tried and untested for the less tried and untested.

Ultimately, the reasons for selecting one particular method over another will be based on local circumstances and personal choice. From our perspective, the need to change in one area was driven by scores on the far left-hand side of the model in Table 4.2, excepting those of quality assurance and workload systems, which were completely alien concepts at the time. Other problems that required resolution included the need to develop staff (for some of whom the only entry on their in service training record was the yearly fire lecture), the need to update clinical practice (the back trolley – oil and spirit and egg white and oxygen were still in use) and the need to improve relationships with all members of the multidisciplinary team. This is not to criticize the abilities of the ward staff. It is a continual source of surprise to us how teams of staff, in spite of appallingly little professional development opportunities in the past, rise to the challenge of change. So what were the factors that helped us push the mark along the work methodology continuum from the left- to the right-hand side of the assessment tool?

Applying change management theory

First (and with the benefit of hindsight) it is worth re-examining the theories of managing change, as all offer some helpful tips. Looking at some of the suggested strategies for managing change, we identified discrete phases recommended in the different theories. We distilled these into the phases of the nursing process as a useful framework for effecting change, which has the added advantage of using terms with which the staff felt comfortable. These were:

- An assessment of the need for change.
- Planning the change process.
- Implementing the changes.
- Evaluating the change.

The process of changing from task allocation to primary nursing is therefore outlined in these four phases.

Phase 1: Assessment

This phase involved our own assessment of the need to change and the 'scanning' of a variety of options from different sources. We also had to devise methods of enabling staff to take part in this process, since, according to the theories, this was a crucial part of effecting the change. Roger's (1979) model refers to the awareness/interest/evaluation stage, which he calls the 'unfreezing' stage. Fretwell's (1985) model shows research findings as the method for gaining insight into the need to change. The problem-solving model uses the recognition of a problem to act as a precursor to change and the change agent model utilizes the diagnosis of the problem as the method of identifying a felt need to change (Tappen, 1989).

The importance of all of these early stages of change management cycles, was in identifying the driving and restraining forces for individuals who were to be involved in the change process. The natural response from most staff when faced with a new idea or threat of change is 'What's in it for me?' This was such a predominant issue that we called it the 'WIIFM' factor. We felt this to be a legitimate response, as we personally would not make any radical change to our professional or private lives without there being a very clear benefit for doing so. These early analyses of the driving and restraining forces at an individual level were therefore crucial if staff were to find their own personal WIIFM factor. Furthermore, we had to ensure that part of our master plan for implementing change included a WIIFM factor for everyone who had the potential to be affected by it. If not, they could present a future restraining force opposing our 'desired level' of Primary Nursing.

Techniques used in the early stages of changing the work methodology
Some of the techniques we found worked best in these early stages were as follows:

Techniques for raising awareness and generating interest
- Arrange regular weekly teaching sessions on different work methodologies and follow these with an open debate on the advantages disadvantages of each.
- Ensure all staff are encouraged to attend the teaching sessions (i.e. untrained staff, medical staff, other professionals and night staff, with rotating times to enable the latter to attend).
- Prepare a summary of teaching and discussion points raised and display these on the notice board for the benefit of staff who missed the session.

- Arrange for staff to visit other units practising primary nursing to hear from peer colleagues about their experiences.
- Send staff to national conferences on Primary Nursing.
- Ensure that staff returning from such study days share their knowledge gained as a result with others, either as an informal feedback session, or a written report.
- Arrange a local conference to enable more staff to attend, with invited outside speakers (this was very cost-effective).
- Circulate journal articles and research findings.
- Start a journal club.

Techniques to define problems and define change goals This was also a powerful method for laying the ground for future changes. The methods we used enabled staff of all grades to change and improve their working environment. For many, it was the first time they had been able to do this, and proved a very strong WIIFM, as they worked on problems that were relevant for them. We found that (as many of the theories earlier suggest) giving staff 'ownership' of such projects was vital to their success.

Techniques used for promoting staff ownership of change
- *Quality circles*. If facilitated properly, these can prove useful in assessing and resolving problems without the usual stresses of more autocratic methods (Kings Fund 1986). Useful questions to start off the initial brainstorming list are:
  (i)   What would you want to change on this ward if you were a patient?
  (ii) What sort of hassles do you encounter regularly that interfere with your work?
  We found the advantage of using this approach was that staff nearly always identified all the problems that we had lost countless nights' sleep over wondering how to raise them without offence or retribution. Also, they often came up with a far better solution to resolve these problems. These tended to 'stick' as they owned the solution and were integral to its implementation. For example, they would check the cardiac arrest trolley daily because they had identified problems at arrests when equipment was missing. The daily check was their own solution to the problem, and was done routinely on their own initiative. Had this been

imposed, there was a danger it would have been done only when we were on duty to coerce them into doing it, and some days the checks would be omitted.

- *Quality assurance tools.* If used appropriately, these can act as extremely useful 'unfreezing' agents. The tools themselves identify problem areas, and these can then be discussed and resolved as a team. In practice, we found the facts and figures in these reports extremely helpful, as they enabled the problems to be presented to staff in an objective way, rather than them perceiving it as Sister getting 'a bee in her bonnet' about a particular problem.

- *Developing a ward philosophy.* A philosophy is:

A statement of the system of beliefs which direct the indivi- · duals in a particular group in the achievement of their purpose. It should be a statement that can be referred to as an explanation of why things are carried out the way they are.

(Cantor, 1973)

The process of developing a ward philosophy proved a useful focus for the team to debate their values and beliefs about what it was we were all trying to achieve in coming to work every day. Brain-storming the question 'Why are we here?' generated many areas for action that had not been considered before. The final statement produced by the team served as a useful anchor point for many of the future discussions, as well as proving a useful 'unfreezer' itself. For example, once the staff identified the concept of individualized patient care as something they wanted to include in their philosophy, we were then able to explore ways in which we were currently fulfilling this objective, and also to highlight areas in which further work needed to be done. This was the big breakthrough we had been waiting for in getting rid of the 'back trolley', when a nursing auxiliary suggested that individual wash bowls for patients would be more 'personal'. This was an item that had proved virtually indestructible to us; even getting the porters to remove it and lock it in the hospital store proved a short-lived victory when, on arriving unannounced at 6 a.m. we found a newly adapted dressing trolley kitted out with all the old ensemble.

We also found it useful to explore the philosophy of Primary Nursing, and ensure that staff understood its principles. We found that some staff had not fully understood these and, in one area, this led to staff stating that they had not been able to 'do' Primary Nursing for several weeks because staff were off sick. They had not understood that changing the work methodology is not purely a matter of changing the way nursing work is allocated, it requires an examination of the values and beliefs that underpin the process of giving care.

The process of raising awareness and defining problems also proved useful for shaping our plans for future phases. Staff suggestions were useful for developing our thoughts and knowledge, and highlighting areas that might prove problematic but that we had not previously considered. As newcomers to the ward, we also used this time to start to build a relationship with the team, using some of the techniques described in the change agent model (Tappen, 1989).

Once the staff had become more aware of the need to review the work methodology, we found it useful to use the assessment tool (Table 4.2) as a rough guide to the status of the factors at the time. The process of allocating scores to these factors generates useful discussion and suggestions which can be incorporated into the planning stage for future action.

Phase 2: Planning

The importance of this initial planning stage cannot be emphasized strongly enough. In our experience, it is extremely difficult to overcome the action-oriented nature of the culture of the nursing profession, and actually allow time for reflective thinking. Nearly all of the initial 'hiccoughs' we experienced when moving on to the next phase could have been avoided if more time and effort had been devoted to Phase 2.

It is also a false premise to assume that things will move faster by moving quickly into Phase 3 (the implementation phase). Inevitably, the time spent sorting out overlooked problems was much greater than the small amount of time that avoiding them would have entailed. For example, in one area, including the domestic staff in the awareness exercises had been overlooked. When the changes were first implemented, this led to subtle alterations in the ward routine, arising from the fact that not all patients were washed at the same time, but at a time to fit in with their plan of care. This meant that the ward was not as accessible for cleaning, as curtains were round the beds, and it completely disrupted the domestics' work schedule. We had not appreciated this problem until the Director of Nursing Services had to intervene to stop industrial action by the frustrated domestics. This created a lot of bad feeling and it was months before the previously harmonious working relationships were restored. Including the domestic staff at the planning stage would have enabled them to identify this problem and use their knowledge of the domestic routine to explore ways around it.

It is for this reason that it is essential to start some of the team building work at this phase. A quick brain-storming session early on, to identify a comprehensive list of everyone who may be affected by the changes, is extremely worthwhile. This list should be referred to constantly when planning the communication factor identified in Table 4.2.

It is also important that, before moving on to the next phase, a comprehensive implementation plan is drawn up, which serves simultaneously to shift the other factors to the desired position in the model in Table 4.2. *before* making any changes to the work methodology. To take the worst possible scenario, if the person 'in charge' of the shift maintains a tight, autocratic control of the staff, the nurse's role is restricted, with an emphasis on technical skills and diffuse accountability, with nurses reluctant to be autonomous for their actions. This will create an appalling working environment, with limited essential nursing equipment and poor geographical design, a 'hit-squad' type quality assurance strategy and a fundamental belief by management that staff dislike work and need close supervision and control. The change agent will use a power coercive approach, the ward will be grossly understaffed, with a predominance of nursing aides, and communications will generally be appalling. In this scenario we can *guarantee* that, even if Florence herself came back to take charge of this ward, there is absolutely no way that stating that 'Primary Nursing will start next Wednesday' would make one iota of difference! This may seem obvious, but it is an approach we have seen in some units.

Phase 3: Implementation

This is the action-oriented phase, during which the work methodology on the ward changes to incorporate the new philosophy. Referring back to the theories of managing change, there are some important key words that are useful to plan and incorporate into this phase. Rogers (1979) refers to a 'trial' at the 'moving' stage of the change process. It is important to remember that this is precisely what the new system is; it is only a trial. Therefore, just as with a clinical trial, there should be a set of measures which can be used as an objective set of indicators for the impact of the new work methodology. This is discussed in more detail under Phase 4. Second, no matter how well the trial has been planned, because change involves individuals it is impossible to control all of the variables that can influence the success of the new method under scrutiny. In our experience, the best advice we can offer is to manage the 'gremlins' as they arise, and keep the implementation plan as flexible as possible. For example, after weeks of planning and discussion, we started on our new routine of a walk-round hand-over, aimed at improving communications and actively involving patients in their plan of care. Despite persevering with various adaptations of the new system, we had eventually to take the whole plan back to the drawing board, due to the trial being an unmitigated disaster. In practice, we found, on this particular ward, that it was taking up to an hour and a half to complete. As the shift overlap was only 15 minutes, understandably it soon became unpopular with staff.

After months of assessment and planning, the first month the changes are implemented can prove extremely stressful. We found that every single thing that went wrong in the early weeks (including being short-staffed due to unforeseen sickness, the mail arriving late, the meals arriving early, three cardiac arrests on one shift and running out of linen) was blamed on the new method of working. It is absolutely crucial that the key change agent takes an extremely objective look at these complaints. Some may well indeed be unforeseen gremlins, and should be managed as above. However, if (as was more often the case) they are the sorts of problems that would have occurred anyway, it is important to take time out with the complainants and review the real cause of the problem. Failure to do this can result in a serious undermining of the new system; to use Pratt's (1982) categories, the 'antagonists' can be so disruptive as to prevent the 'acquiescers' from settling into the new way of working.

Finding physical things to do to implement these changes (so far only abstract concepts, good intentions and innovative ideas) to enable them to become part of established practice is something we found lacking in the theoretical textbooks on the subject. What we present below is therefore a 'top tips' list, which, in our experience, were important in changing the work methodology on the ward.

Top tip 1: Include actions and target dates on the implementation plan.

Don't set wishy washy actions and targets or enormous unachievable goals; remember, if you are going to eat an elephant, it is best done one bite at a time. Small, specific targets are much easier to achieve, manage and evaluate. Review these regularly, ensure staff are assigned actions complete them and modify them if necessary.

Top tip 2: Undertake a radical review of the off-duty rota

First, the skill and grade mix of staff needs to be examined. Make any staff changes, new appointments, changes in shift times, etc. Allow enough time to elapse to allow staff to adapt to the alterations. Second, change the format of the off-duty to one done in teams. This involves:

- Selecting the teams.
- Allocating patients to the teams.
- Rostering the teams.

Selecting the teams When dividing the staff up into teams, the first decision that needs to be taken is on how many teams there should be. A greater number of teams will reduce the different number of nurses that will care for a particular patient, which can be an advantage in promoting continuity of care. The big disadvantage is that preparing the duty rota becomes even more difficult as there is less flexibility to incorporate off-duty and holiday requests. Discuss the options with the staff, it is important that they understand the implications. As a rough guide, for an average 26-bed general adult ward, up to full staffing establishment, we would recommend two or three teams. Units with a higher ratio of trained to untrained staff (e.g. coronary care or intensive care) could possibly manage up to four teams.

The next decision is to determine which staff go into which team. Broadly speaking, it is wise to ensure that all teams have roughly similar grade mix, with equal numbers of whole-time equivalents. Having drawn up the initial list (e.g. each team will have 1 G or F grade, 2 E grade, 1.5 D grade, 2 C grade, and 3 A grades, with a B grade 'floating ' in the role of ward auxiliary) it is then necessary to assign individual staff members to a team. An excellent way to do this is include it in a team-building session, where staff can explore the skills needed to make the team effective and be involved in selecting the teams. Done in this way, it prevents the speculation as to why 'X' is in one team and 'Y' in another that inevitably arises if a list of two teams appears on the notice board.

Personality issues inevitably creep into the selection process, but it is best to allocate a broad range of similar skills to both teams, rather than rely on the personal preferences of individuals. It is also worth pointing out to staff who want to be in the same team as the colleagues they mix with socially that, for most of the time, they will be rostered on the opposite shift.

The one exception to this 'rule of equals' advice is if it has been opted to assign different workloads (e.g. all high dependency patients) to a particular team. In our experience to do this on a long-term basis causes a large amount of ill-feeling between teams, and is not recommended. Alternatives include rotating the teams every few months and swapping 50% of each team around every 4 months to prevent feudalism building up.

Allocating patients to the teams The process of selecting which patient should be cared for by which team can be influenced by a number of factors:

- *The workload*. Whichever method of patient allocation is chosen, once the initial split has been made it is important to ensure that, as new patients are admitted, the workload for each team remains roughly equal. This can be achieved by assessing the workload of each team, the dependency of the patient on admission, and assigning the patient accordingly. This should be done by the ward co-ordinator.

- *Specific nursing skills.* As a result of the team-building and staff development programmes, many of the staff develop specialist skills and knowledge, which are worth considering when allocating patients to a team. Hence it is logical to allocate the patient with an acute myocardial infarction to the team with the nurse who has finished the CCU course; the patient with uncontrolled diabetes to the team with the nurse who is carrying out research on the effect of a new teaching programme for diabetics, etc. This not only benefits the patient, it also encourages staff to apply their nursing knowledge and to share this with other team members.

- *Ward geography.* It is worth examining the ward geography when allocating patients to a team of nurses. Having patients dotted around all over the ward in various locations can fragment the teams' time, and mean they cannot easily observe patients in their care. On an old Nightingale-style ward, we found the easiest way was to divide the ward in half, with all one team's patients down the left-hand side of the ward and all the other team's patients down the right. After the initial furniture-moving session, by allocating patients to a team on admission they automatically went into the correct team's bed. It also made the daily SHO ward round, drug administration and meal times easier; the team leader from one team went up one side of the ward and the team leader from the other side took over half way round.

  In our experience, having beds allocated randomly to a team creates chaos on a ward round. It fragments the nurses' time, as they continually have to 'hang around' for the Doctors to reach their patients, and the medical staff found it confusing and disruptive, particularly if one nurse disappeared and the other failed to materialize. Bays can be similarly divided, either as one whole bay to a team, or splitting the bay in half so nurses from opposite teams can cover each others' meal breaks.

- *Consultant-based teams.* Originally we threw our hands up in horror, as the whole suggestion seemed to ooze with subservience to the medical profession. We were wary of promoting the idea of the Consultant having 'his' or 'her' nurse. However, it is only fair to report that in one area with two

Consultants, each with roughly equal workloads, this greatly influenced the ease of passage to the new work methodology. It also greatly improved the relationship between nursing and medical staff, and the latter showed great commitment in contributing to the in-service training programmes for staff. This led eventually to protocols being written on topics ranging from pressure sores (prevention and treatment) to cardiac arrest. It made the Consultants' ward rounds easier to incorporate into the nurses' work plan, as the team leader could go round all the patients at once, and make an active contribution to the round.

Gaining the support from the medical staff was a major coup in terms of gaining recognition from other professionals (and some members of our own profession) and we recommend this as a worthwhile venture to be encouraged. It also led to greater continuity of care, as the Consultant would ring the ward if there was a patient in clinic for admission in the future. This enabled a member of the team to go and meet the patient, and offer them the chance to ask questions or visit the ward.

- *Personal preference or previous admission.* On some occasions, patients were allocated to a particular team irrespective of the workload. This would either be because the patient had been on the ward previously and had been cared for by one team, or at the express wish of specific team members. This was usually as the patient had specific nursing problems in which certain team members had expertise or interest. On very rare occasions, there were personality clashes between a patient and member of staff. It is important to remember this is not a problem resulting directly from the new system, but the system can exacerbate the situation, as the patient is allocated on a regular basis to the same member of staff. The causes for the difficulty need to be explored and resolved on an individual basis. However, allocating the patient to another team or moving the nurse temporarily to another team are both viable options, with appropriate counselling and support.

Rostering the teams Prior to actually attempting to compile the new team off-duty, it is worth reflecting on the following two questions, which, with the benefit of hindsight, would have saved us a few grey hairs!

When is the best time of to introduce the new system? Obviously, this is influenced by the progress made in preparing all the other factors. However, if starting from scratch in developing a timetable of change, we recommend that all other factors are planned with a view to starting the new rota system in April. This is not such an 'Alice-In-Wonderland'-type reply as first appears. In all NHS hospitals the current working year runs from the beginning of April, as does the staff holiday year. It can be appreciated that there are major advantages in starting the new teams before any annual leave is booked. This prevents the situation where three staff are off on leave on one team (making it impossible to cover the shifts) and all the other team is present. If it is impractical to introduce the system in April, it is worth selecting the teams at this time (even though the off-duty will not be done in teams for several months) and considering them when staff start to request annual leave.

Alternatively, if it is already too far into the year, and the time seems right to start team off-duty, then introducing previously booked annual leave as another criterion to consider when selecting staff for a team can overcome the problem. Failure to do this results in poor morale among staff, either because they are asked to change their holidays, or asked to swap teams to cover holiday shifts. This latter option completely undermines the whole philosophy, particularly if it happens on a regular basis.

It is also a good strategic move to make sure that the staff who have demonstrated enthusiasm and commitment are not on holiday during the first trial weeks. The most senior nurses should most certainly not be. If there are still any remaining 'laggards' in spite of all the preparation, it is certainly worth checking when they are on holiday (although this needs to be done extremely discreetly). In our experience, if they come back to a system that their peers demonstrate can work, and show commitment to, peer pressure usually encourages them to at least give it a try. Also, it gives the other staff a bit more space during the early days to overcome their own anxieties concerning the change and enables them to gain confidence in the new methods. They are then more able to give the required support and encouragement that is needed to help these individuals, many of whom are motivated by fear of the unknown.

Do we have an effective method for compiling off-duty rotas? In our case, the answer was a resounding 'no'. Off-duty compilation had always been a well-kept trade secret, with Sister disappearing into the office for hours on end, only to come out for brief periods of hair pulling, or to ask if you'd really mind working a 150 hour week after all! At the end of it all, it would miraculously be pinned to the wall, in time for everyone to ask if she would mind if they just swapped the one shift here and . . .

We started off, as no doubt many others do, with what can only be referred to as 'social' off-duty. We tried to please everyone and give them not only their holidays and requested days off, but shift preferences as well. Invariably that left us personally with the worst possible off-duty, and, looking at it realistically, staff not always on at the times they were most needed. We were also making a rod for our own backs, some staff abused the good will, and the preference quickly became the norm, with considerable resentment shown if these were not granted. We recommend the following steps as a useful cure for 'social off-duty' syndrome:

- *Step 1.* It is imperative to examine the workload trends on the ward. Take the last month's figures and plot them on a graph. This in itself is a useful exercise, as it immediately allows trends to be seen. In the example in Figure 4.4, it is easy to see that the workload is reduced markedly at the weekend, and rises steadily throughout the week. This is a pattern typically seen on surgical wards. Different trends will be established on other types of ward, with areas such as acute medical wards showing seemingly more random distribution; in these areas it is necessary to review patterns over a much longer period of time. This exercise often shows marked seasonal variation.

    Our first introduction to such seemingly obvious information led to some serious mocking of the whole notion of such workload dependency tools, after all (we cried) why spend all this time and money working out something that all good nurses could tell you anyway? If this is indeed the response, we recommend the following exercise.

    Under the graph for the monthly workload; plot the total hours worked by staff for each of the shifts for that same month (as shown in Figure 4.4). Does the 'staff hours' pattern

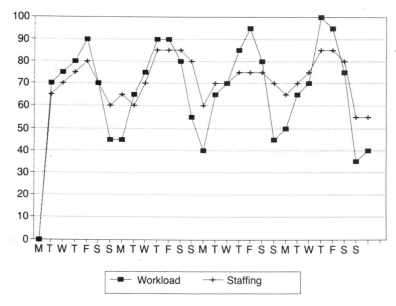

Figure 4.4 Workload dependency analysis pattern on a surgical ward.

match the workload? Ours certainly did not and, from experience in implementing such tools in a considerable number of other units, this is not a unique phenomenon. We had fallen into the classic trap we were desperately trying to change – we weren't putting our knowledge into practice. In one instance, despite the typical 'surgical ward' type pattern shown (Figure 4.4), there was only a limited staff reduction on some weekends, and in no way did this mirror the drastic fall in workload.

Similarly, the marked rise in workload in the middle of the week was not matched by a corresponding rise in staff. At the other extreme, on a medical ward, the more random pattern indicates that it is much harder to predict fluctuations in workload. It is therefore logical to maintain a fairly constant number of staff throughout the week. In fact, we found that numbers were traditionally reduced at weekends, with random fluctuations throughout the week.

- *Step 2*. Discuss these anomalies openly with staff, and invite suggestions on how to resolve these difficulties. In our experience, they often come up with really good suggestions for improvement. Second, we found (to our cost) that radical off-duty alterations are one of the biggest restraining forces for any change. If staff can see the WIIFM factor in matching off-duty with workload, and feel their suggestions are acted on, this can be a powerful driving force. We identified the following WIIFM's:

(i) It would benefit staff, as the periods where the workload was higher than the number of nurse hours available were extremely stressful.

(ii) It would benefit patients, as inevitably being under-staffed meant certain aspects of patient care were neglected.

(iii) In some instances, it meant more weekends off for staff.

(iv) It meant less overtime, the most common cause being trained staff staying late at the end of understaffed shifts to write care plans.

(v) It was generally felt to be more fair.

- *Step 3.* Off-duty needs to be planned to match predicted workload. This needs to take account of current trends and any known variables that will affect these in the next month, for example theatre lists cancelled due to medical staff holidays, local events such as half marathons, etc. This may sound obvious, but this occurred a significant number of times in our respective units. Checking with medical records or the Consultants for the former proved worthwhile, as it enabled us to run study days for staff, or allow extra staff leave.

After much trial and error, we have found that the following 10-step method of compiling rotas to match nursing workload works well:

(i) Take the blank rota and list the names of both the teams, one above the other, with extra rows labelled to calculate the total trained staff for each team, the total numbers for each team per shift and the grand total of staff on duty at the bottom; as shown on the far left-hand side of Table 4.3.

(ii) By each name, write the grade of staff and the total number of shifts worked per week (e.g. full time = five shifts, with the exception of night duty, which is discussed below).

(iii) In the column labelled 'total shifts available,' write the

Table 4.3 Off-duty compilation for team nursing (1)

	Contracted full shifts	Monday	Tuesday	Wednesday	Thursday	Friday	Saturday	Sunday
Yellow team								
Karen (G)	5							
Mary (E)	5	A/L	A/L	A/L	A/L	A/L	D.O.	D.O.
Bridget (E)	3							
Barbara (D)	5							
Katherine (C)	5							
Total shifts av.	18	1/1	2/1	2/2	2/1	1/1	1/1	1/1
Pat (A)	5							
Carol (A)	4							
Joe (A)	5							
Total shifts av.	14	1/1	1/1	1/1	1/1	1/1	1/1	1/1
Totals (a.m. and p.m.)		2/2	3/2	3/3	3/2	2/2	2/2	2/2
Orange team								
Phil (F)	5							
Robin (E)	4							
Sheila (E)	4							
Judy (D)	4							
Kathy (C)	5	A/L	A/L	A/L	A/L	A/L	D/O	D/O
Total shifts av.	17	1/1	2/1	2/1	2/1	1/1	1/1	1/1
Brian (A)	5							
Kim (A)	5		A/L	A/L	A/L			
Zoe (A)	4							
Total shifts av.	12	1/1	1/1	1/1	1/1	1/1	1/	1/
Totals (a.m. and p.m.)		2/2	3/2	3/2	3/2	2/2	2/1	2/1
Grand total		4/4	6/4	6/5	6/4	4/4	4/3	4/3
Joyce		9–5	9–5	9–5	9–5	9–5	D.O.	D.O.

A/L, annual leave; av., available; D.O., day off.

total number of shifts available for rostering that week, i.e. excluding all annual leave, bank holidays, maternity leave and notified sickness. For example, in Table 4.3 trained staff in the Yellow team would normally have 23 shifts, but five of those are unavailable as Mary is on holiday, leaving 18 available for rostering. Complete this exercise for the trained and untrained staff in each team.

(iv)   The minimum number of trained staff shifts required to ensure one trained member is on every shift is 14 (i.e. seven early shifts and seven late shifts to cover Monday to Sunday.) In the example shown, the Yellow team has 18 shifts available, which means there are four shifts free to be allocated when the ward is most busy. As the workload is known to be heaviest on Tuesday mornings, all day Wednesday and Thursday mornings, these four shifts are rostered to correspond with demand. Hence the 'total shifts available' column for Tuesday, Wednesday and Thursday shows 2/1 2/2 and 2/1, meaning that two staff are needed for the early shift on Tuesday, and are on the late; and so on. Complete this exercise for the trained and untrained 'Total shifts available' rows for both teams.

(v)   Add the total numbers of staff on each team per shift. In the example shown, Yellow team has 1/1 trained and 1/1 untrained staff rostered for Monday, giving the 'Totals' (a.m. and p.m.) as 2/2, i.e. two staff on the early shift and two on the late shift.

(vi)   Sum the grand total of staff on duty, shown in the penultimate column of Table 4.4. Hence on Monday, Yellow team has two staff on an early and two on a late, as does the orange team, giving a grand total of four on the early and four on the late.

(vii)   Pencil in all off-duty requests (shown as 'r' in Table 4.4).

(viii) Allocate the correct number of days off for all staff. Using the trained staff in Yellow team as an example, it can be seen from Table 4.4 that this is relatively simple. On Monday, two staff are needed, one for each shift. Above these numbers are four staff available for work. Two can therefore have the day off, and Katherine has requested it. On Wednesday, a total of four staff is

Table 4.4 Off-duty compilation for team nursing (2)

	Contracted full shifts	Monday	Tuesday	Wednesday	Thursday	Friday	Saturday	Sunday
Yellow team								
Karen (G)	5	L	E*	E†	D.O.	D.O.	L	E
Mary (E)	5	A/L	A/L	A/L	A/L	A/L	D.O.	D.O.
Bridget (E)	3	D.O.	L	E	E	D.O.	D.O.	D.O.
Barbara (D)	5	E	E	L	L	E	D.O.	D.O.
Katherine (C)	5	D.O.[r]	D.O.[r]	L	E	L	E	L
Total shifts av.	18	1/1	2/1	2/2	2/1	1/1	1/1	1/1
Pat (A)	5	D.O.	D.O.	L	E	L	E	L
Carol (A)	4	L	E	D.O.	D.O.	D.O.	L	E
Joe (A)	5	E	L	E	L	E	D.O.	D.O.
Total shifts av.	14	1/1	1/1	1/1	1/1	1/1	1/1	1/1
Totals (a.m. and p.m.)		2/2	3/2	3/3	3/2	2/2	2/2	2/2
Orange team								
Phil (F)	5	E	E*	E	L[r]	E	D.O.[r]	D.O.[r]
Robin (E)	4	D.O.	D.O.	L	E	D.O.	E[r]	L[r]
Sheila (E)	4	D.O.	L	E	E	L[r]	D.O.	D.O.
Judy (D)	4	L	E	D.O.	D.O.	D.O.	L	E
Kathy (C)	5	A/L	A/L	A/L	A/L	A/L	D.O.	D.O.
Total shifts av.	17	1/1	2/1	2/1	2/1	1/1	1/1	1/1
Brian (A)	5	D.O.[r]				D.O.[r]	D.O.	D.O.
Kim (A)	5		A/L	A/L	A/L			
Zoe (C)	4					E[r]		
Total shifts av.	12	1/1	1/1	1/1	1/1	1/1	1/	1/
Totals (a.m. and p.m.)		2/2	3/2	3/2	3/2	2/2	2/1	2/1
Grand total		4/4	6/4	6/5	6/4	4/4	4/3	4/3
Joyce		9–5	9–5	9–5	9–5	9–5	D.O.	D.O.

A/L, annual leave; av., available; D.O., day off; E, early; L, late; [r], request; *, sisters' meeting 11 a.m.; †, teaching a.m.

needed to cover the workload, and there are four staff above these numbers who are available to work. No days off can therefore be given (make sure to scan across the week at regular intervals to ensure not to allocate days off to staff who may have requested days off at the end of the week).

(ix)   As far as possible, pencil in early shifts before, and late shifts after, days off.

(x)   Fill in any remaining blanks with the required shifts, taking account of staff duties on the previous day. For example, referring back to Table 4.4, Yellow team, untrained staff, on Monday (which is still incomplete). There are two blank spaces, and two staff are needed to work, one an early, one a late. As Brian was off the previous weekend, and Zoe on holiday on Tuesday, it makes sense to give Brian the late, and Zoe the early. Complete the whole off duty in this way. Remember, when allocating the early and late shifts for trained staff in the second team, to keep one eye on the rostered shifts of the first team to ensure a good skill mix overall, i.e. not both Sisters on the late shift and the D and C grades on the early.

The 10-step method can be used to compile an off-duty that matches nursing workload for more complex rotas. For ease of explanation, the rota shown in Tables 4.3 and 4.4 has been kept as straightforward as possible. However, this method can be used for more complex rotas if necessary. Night-duty staff can be integrated into the rota where internal rotation is practised. Include the names on the rota, and where the 'total shifts available' and 'grand total' columns appear, a third figure will be included in the totals, which will be the night-duty staff. For example, the grand total column for Monday could read 4/4/3, if three night staff were required. It is easier if the night shifts are rostered first. Part-time staff can also be used with this method, the number of shifts or part shifts should be indicated by their names, and incorporated into the rota in the same way.

Compiling off-duty using the 10-step method is beneficial if the teams progress to the stage where it is appropriate to commence Primary Nursing. Each team will have a number of Primary and Associate Nurses. The Primary Nurse will have a caseload of patients, and other Primary Nurses or Associate Nurses in that team will carry out the prescribed care when he or she is off duty. This helps maintain the continuity of care, as fewer different nurses will care for the patient. A general tip worth noting is to wind down the caseload for the Primary Nurses prior to their holidays. A week or so before (depending on the average length of patient stay on the ward) it is advisable not to allocate them any new patients, and roster them to act as Associate Nurses instead. There is little point in them taking a new patient and planning care if they are not on duty for two weeks. The ward co-ordinator for each shift can be highlighted on the rota.

Top tip 3: Introduce team nursing first
Unless the initial assessment scores of the ward are well to the right of the assessment model, we would strongly recommend that team nursing is implemented first. This allows a gentle 'weaning in' period and makes the final changes to Primary Nursing much smoother, as many of the initial teething problems can be resolved.

Top tip 4: Avoid Sister/Charge Nurses taking on a Primary Nurse Caseload
In the early stages, the Primary Nurses require a lot of support, best provided by the Sister/Charge Nurse, who can act as a role model and adviser; this is difficult if he or she is carrying a caseload. Acting as Associate Nurse also gives them the opportunity to evaluate the Primary Nurse informally in the clinical setting. Once the new methodology is well established, it is often possible for them to manage a small caseload.

Top tip 5: Devise a system to communicate the patient's team/Primary Nurse to patients and staff.
There is nothing more disheartening for a Primary Nurse or Team Leader than to have relatives, medical staff and other professionals continually asking if they can speak to Sister about their caseload patients. Some of this can be alleviated by a good communication exercise in the planning stage. Ongoing solutions we found useful in helping alleviate this problem were as follows:

- An explanation of the role of Primary Nurse to patients and relatives on admission.
- A notice-board with an explanation of the work methodology on the ward, with photographs of the staff.
- Labelling the beds with the name or colour of the Team, and, if appropriate, the Primary Nurse.
- Patient information booklets, explaining the system of patient allocation, with the name of their Team or Primary Nurse.
- Small business cards for relatives with the ward telephone number and the name of the Team or Primary Nurse to ask for.
- The Sister/Charge Nurse continually referring enquiries back to the Primary Nurse.
- Clear name badges for staff, with names on the background colour corresponding to their team.

Top tip 6: Review the systems used for nurse handover
In our experience, the length of handover increases proportionally with the knowledge the nurses have of their patients. However, under the new system, there is little to be gained from an hour's monologue on patients staff will see little, or nothing of for the whole shift. At the other extreme we have also experienced difficulties if a patient calls us over and we know nothing about him or her, or if there is a telephone enquiry and the Team Leader or Primary Nurse is at tea. Strategies that we found useful to overcome these problems include:

- A brief, factual handover to all staff on all patients by the Ward Co-ordinator, followed by a more detailed report from the previous shift's Primary Nurse or Team Leader to the oncoming staff on their allocated patients only.
- Reviewing where handovers take place, and the methods used. These can exclude the patient completely (i.e. take place in the office or nurse's station), include the patient partially (i.e. a brief report elsewhere, followed by a bedside handover), or be patient-led (i.e. the patients explain to oncoming nurses the aspects of care that concern oncoming staff, with supplementary information from the nurse handing over).

There is no 'ideal' method, it is largely dependent on the type of patients, the geography on the ward and the preference of the staff. One word of warning about bedside handovers. We have found these beneficial when the patient is keen to, and given the opportunity to, participate in handing over to a small number of staff. At the other extreme, a large number of nurses at the bottom of the bed talking about, rather than to the patient, can be distressing for the patient, and undermines the whole philosophy of individualized, holistic care.

Top tip 7: Ensure the new work methodology will also work on night duty

Part of the planning stage involves including night staff in discussions on the new work methodology; the philosophy is seriously undermined if the ward reverts to task allocation between 9 p.m. and 7 a.m. Often, the staffing levels at night make it more difficult (although still possible) to maintain Team/Primary Nursing. Most wards have only two trained nurses on duty at night and for this reason it is often easier to run two teams than three. The night nurses are then allocated to a team in the same way as the rest of the staff. The practicalities of permanent night staff being Primary Nurses need to be explored by the team. From our experience, it can prove problematic, as the relatives and other professionals are not generally seen at night, and, ideally, the patient is asleep for most of it. However, they can easily fulfil the role of Associate Nurses.

Top tip 8: Set clear requirements for all the staff roles

One of the biggest problems we encountered when changing the work methodology was that staff were often unclear what was expected of them. This can largely be addressed in the planning stage for Factor 3, which examines the role of the nurse at differing ends of a continuum. Role definition may require continual re-enforcement during the implementation phase.

A common problem we encountered when roles were not clear was the changing of the plan of care by staff other than the Team Leader or Primary Nurse, either by other team members, by associate nurses or by the person who, under the old system, would have been 'in charge'. Another difficulty when roles were misunderstood was that other professionals tended to look for the latter person, rather than the nurse caring for the patient, for information. These problems can often be resolved by gentle reminders and re-enforcement of the new roles. In other cases, it can be the result of deliberate subversion of the new system, and this needs to be tackled in the most appropriate way, immediately.

Purpose of the 'top tips'
These tips are not presented as an exhaustive list to guarantee the successful implementation of the new work methodology. We have identified those areas that, with the benefit of hindsight, were, or could have been, instrumental in taking our master plan off the notice board and putting it into practice.

Although the changes are presented as four discrete phases, namely assessment, planning, implementation and evaluation, in practice, the margins between these were very blurred. This is particularly the case between phases 3 (implementation) and 4 (planning), where the certain aspects of evaluation will, by necessity, be started early on in phase 3. These will be now be examined.

Phase 4: The evaluation phase for introducing the new work methodology

Referring back to the theories of change, the end stage in Fretwell's (1985) model is 'recording the findings of the change'. Rogers (1979) offers the option of the adaptation being accepted or rejected. Cuba and Clark (1978) refer in their taxonomy to the institutionalization of the change. The major difficulty experienced by many authors attempting to evaluate the impact of the new work methodology is in determining what criteria to measure. A further difficulty is that, often, the adaptation or rejection of the new methodology bears no relation to the findings of the study. In one area (Pembrey, 1989) in spite of demonstrable advantages of Primary Nursing, the unit was forced to close. Other studies (Shulkar and Turner: Ventura et al., in Macdonald, 1988) show no clear relationship between the introduction of Primary Nursing and improved patient outcomes, and yet persist with the new work methodology. Although there is a growing body of literature on Primary Nursing, only a small proportion of it is research based, with one author arguing that many of these studies were seriously methodologically flawed (Giovannetti, 1986). One claim made by some studies, and many subjective reports, is that Primary Nursing increases job satisfaction for the nurses (Reed 1988).

This could explain the persistence of implementing this approach in the absence of other more concrete benefits, again highlighting the strength of the 'WIIFM' factor in driving change. These findings are all relevant to the application of change theories to clinical practice, as many appear to assume that need to change is based on a logical, rational approach to decision making. In practice, it would appear often not to be the case.

It is extremely easy, coming back from conferences full of glowing anecdotes on the benefits of Primary Nursing, to launch enthusiastically into a change programme, without giving any thought on how to evaluate its benefits. From experience, there are five important reasons why this should not be allowed to happen.

- Sooner or later, when resources become tight, it is inevitable that budget-tied managers are going to ask for evidence that this approach is better than any other. Without it, the skill mix on the ward may be altered, which prevents the continuation of the new method of work allocation. This is a very real threat with the phasing-in of Health Care Assistants.
- Other professional groups who may be more cynical about the new approach will also be looking for evidence of its benefits. Clear indicators of improvement are more powerful weapons than subjective reports.
- As a profession striving to be research based, we have a professional duty to evaluate the impact of our care-giving.
- These changes take so long to implement, it is often difficult to remember how much progress has been made. Setting bench marks along the way can help indicate to staff their achievements to date.
- It is extremely useful to staff from other units visiting those further ahead than theirs on the road to changing to Primary Nursing if they can be given clear measures of what can be achieved. This is useful for setting their own action plans, but also in convincing more sceptical staff and managers in their own units.

Research is regarded by many ward-based nurses as something that is inherently difficult, and best left to the academics. Realistically, the chances of many ward-based staff being given the time and resources to carry out a full-scale research study into the benefits of the new system are limited. However, one should not preclude this option, and for many nurses on post-graduate degree programmes, this is a fertile and worthwhile area.

If the above is not an option and evaluation is not possible, we would strongly agree with the following sentiments:

> The changes involved in primary nursing are so great and potentially far reaching that the question 'Is primary nursing better than team nursing or patient allocation or task alloca-tion?' is probably one we should not be trying to answer. We would probably get further if we were to look at changes in particular aspects of practice, or the effectiveness of the same practice under different modalities.   (*MacGuire, 1989*)

Again, we return to the reflection that if you have to eat an elephant it is best to do it one bite at a time. Inviting your col-leagues to share it with you is an even more effective way to do it; and can help avoid the psychological indigestion that occurs when biting off a project that is too big to chew. The first task in setting up a comprehensive set of evaluation tools to examine particular aspects of practice is therefore to raise the interest of the ward staff and other colleagues in the research and to equip them in the skills to do it. We found the following methods useful in helping us achieve this aim:

- Start a journals club.
- Send staff on research courses, study days and conferences, and allow them to share knowledge gained with other staff.
- Include a small-scale research study as an objective in staff appraisals.
- Allow staff time to attend local or regional research interest groups.
- Find out which members of staff in other areas, and in other professions, have ongoing studies, an interest in research or specialist skills such as statistical or computer knowledge, and encourage them to contribute wherever possible.
- If the hospital has a quality assurance team, contact them and see what tools they have on offer. They may carry out some form of audit for you.

- Contact the medical audit group and see if they have any resources or expertise that may help. Find out if they have any on-going audits that can be used as a baseline measure (e.g. infection rates, average length of stay, etc.).
- Contact the local universities and colleges for information on courses and establish links with the research and health studies departments. They can often offer advice and support, and may have post-graduates looking for access into clinical areas to research a subject that could also be useful for evaluation purposes.
- Contact the Regional Health Authority and find out if any funds are available for locally organized research.

Following these preliminary initiatives, the serious business of establishing criteria for measurement begins. At this stage, it is worth referring to the original philosophy and aims and objectives for criteria for measurement. If these include statements such as 'increased patient satisfaction' and 'improved job satisfaction', it is worth reviewing the literature to find appropriate 'off the shelf' valid patient satisfaction or staff attitude survey tools. A wide variety is available, and it is an alternative to developing one from scratch.

The use of patient care studies can be another useful method of evaluation, albeit more subjective. These can act as valuable material to form the basis of peer review. This involves giving staff 'time out' to discuss certain aspects of nursing care in a supportive setting and to review the rationale for their prescribed plan of care. This encourages professional development and sharing of clinical expertise. The use of a professional journal can be another useful method for tracking the professional development of staff.

On a broader level, it is also worth reviewing the quality assurance tools outlined in Chapter 3. These are usually well validated, relatively easy to apply and provide useful bench marks that are easily replicable for comparison at regular intervals.

It is then worthwhile to seek out the special interest areas of staff, and support them in developing small-scale research projects into these. For example, the staff with an interest in wound care could record the incidence of wound infections and pressure sore developments as a very simple project, feeding the results back to the clinical audit meeting at regular intervals. As confidence grows, they can conduct literature reviews into different modes of treatment for these complications and, in conjunction with the multidisciplinary team, draw up treatment protocols and evaluate the effectiveness of these.

Another approach worth considering at this stage, is to calculate comparative cost savings as a result of new practices. For example, a pilot study may show a 96% decrease in pressure sore formation in at-risk patients as a result of using a new type of mattress. Using data such as cost of treatment and cost of extended length of hospital stay, it is possible to estimate the current cost to the hospital in treating pressure sores (Hibbs, 1988). Ninety Six per cent of the estimated cost of treatment is a powerful tool when arguing for the funding for extending the use of the mattresses. In our experience, managers really start to take notice when schemes are presented to them along with this kind of financial information.

This leads on to the next important point, namely that different individuals involved in the change (e.g. nurses, patients, doctors, managers and other staff groups) all have different 'success' criteria by which they will measure any new innovation.

Using a 'pluralistic evaluation' i.e. one that considers 'success criteria' as defined by all the individuals (referred to as 'stakeholders') who have the potential to affect, or be affected by the change is an approach recommended worthy of consideration. (Smith and Cantley, 1985). In our experience, this has several advantages.

First, determining the general expectations of these key stakeholders *before* implementing change offers the change agent enormous potential to incorporate these criteria into the objectives for the project, and therefore increase the likelihood of it being regarded as a 'success' by all. For example, on a semi-structured interview to determine what different groups of 'stakeholders' would regard as success criteria for Primary Nursing, one may ascertain that the patients would expect to get to know one particular nurse better, which would make it easier for them to approach him or her with difficult problems or anxieties. The nurses may cite increased job satisfaction and personal development for staff as key criteria, whilst the doctors may expect improved discharge teaching and planning, and reduced patient non-compliance to treatment. Exploring ways to fulfil these criteria, and ways of measuring them, is therefore a worthwhile exercise.

Second, in terms of predicting the likelihood of the change being accepted, and, to use Lewin's concept of 're-freezing' at the new level, it is worth reflecting on the power politics prevalent in the area for change. The pluralist theory of power argues that power is distributed widely among different groups, and that all are able to exert some influence, although this may vary between the groups. Conversely, the elitist approach argues that certain groups are predominant over others. Alford (1975) argues that the medical profession is the dominant group within the health service. Stocking (1984) found in her study that neither of the two theories exemplified the whole truth about power in the NHS, but both were useful, particularly in providing insights into how innovations develop and why particular individuals become involved and why particular outcomes occurred.

In summary, to ignore specific stakeholders' criteria for success restricts the change agent's understanding of potentially valuable insights that may assist with the change process. They may have valid objectives, previously unconsidered, that will strengthen the validity of the evaluation. Even if these criteria are regarded by other stakeholders as questionable, it is worth remembering that this is what these individuals expect to see if they are to judge the new work methodology a success. If it is perceived by them to be a failure, they can become restraining forces opposing the proposed change. If, in addition, they are a group with a monopoly of power in local decision making, they can veto the change completely. This has already happened in one unit that had introduced Primary Nursing successfully and was forced to close (Pembrey and Punton, 1990).

There is no prescriptive method on how to change the work methodology in a ward. General pointers and frameworks can be offered to help, but the key to its success will be in applying and adapting these into an approach that is locally acceptable to all stakeholders.

Third, developing a tool based on pluralistic criteria, and using it with the different stakeholders at regular intervals throughout the change process, allows the researcher to compare the opinions of the different groups. This is valuable both in terms of tracking progress, and to identify stakeholders who may feel the change is not beneficial. This can act as a precursor to discussions on problem areas and effective solutions. It also ensures that groups with significantly smaller numbers do not have their viewpoint lost in average scores from much larger groups.

Finally, this approach has the advantage of being dynamic and flexible enough to adapt to the change process. Typically, as any new innovation (this one included) develops, the success criteria tend to change. For example, we earlier quoted our experience of the failure of a walk-round handover. To continue to use criteria such as 'Does the Primary Nurse receive a bedside handover?' would therefore be inappropriate. This is a danger when using some of the commercially available quality assurance tools described in Chapter 3.

Another specific research approach that offers potential for evaluating change by integrating the role of researcher as change agent is that of action research (Webb, 1989). In practice, we have found it extremely difficult to establish a traditional clinical trial, complete with control group, to measure the impact of a differing work methodology. Finding a matched control group, with similar wards (i.e. patients, staff, environment and numerous other variables) is virtually impossible. Even if this hurdle could be overcome, it is practically impossible to prove that any improvement in patient outcome was due solely to the work methodology, as these will also be dependent on inputs from the other members of the multidisciplinary team, the patient, the environment and numerous other factors. Action research offers an interesting alternative to more traditional research methods in offering a different approach to some of these methodological problems.

We see evaluation as an integral part of the change process, as an activity that is on-going and proactive, rather than reactive. The results should be utilized to monitor and develop the objectives of the change process, and methods used should be flexible enough to do this. It is advisable to pick several initial key measures, as although it may be tempting to go for a quick, baseline audit using an off-the-shelf quality assurance tool, these are not intended to audit the breadth of wide ranging areas that changing the work methodology has the potential to impact.

The four stages of managing change outlined above are (like the nursing process) a cyclical process, with the evaluation being used as the basis for future action plans and modification of the current one.

SUMMARY

This chapter has two central foci, namely the process of change and the introduction of Primary Nursing into the clinical setting. Implicit in these two themes was link made at the beginning of the chapter between both of these factors as offering potential mechanisms for improving the quality of care. The theories of change management were explored and developed in an attempt to gain insight into the change process that might assist us as practising nurses to develop a comprehensive approach to manage the transition to Primary Nursing. Drawing on these theories of change management, four phases were identified as beneficial in managing this transition. These were:

- Phase 1: the assessment phase.
- Phase 2: the planning phase.
- Phase 3: the implementation phase.
- Phase 4: the evaluation phase.

Strategies were then suggested for each of these phases, based on our own experiences in implementing Primary Nursing in a clinical setting, which we had found to be effective.

However, our own experience had also identified a number of other factors that required consideration if the change to Primary Nursing was to be achieved. Drawing on some of the change theories, an assessment tool was introduced (and shown in Figure 4.5). The first two of these factors; namely change management theory, and work methodology have now been explored fully. The other factors identified were:

- Factor 3 – nursing role.
- Factor 4 – nurse accountability.
- Factor 5 – environment.
- Factor 6 – workload systems.
- Factor 7 – leadership style.
- Factor 8 – communications.
- Factor 9 – quality assurance.

Factor 9, (quality assurance) has been outlined in Chapter 3. Chapter 5 is devoted to exploring the remaining factors, and their influence on achieving the aim of Primary Nursing. The final section at the end of Chapter 5 offers some suggestions for integrating all of these factors into an overall plan to ensure that this aim is realized.

REFERENCES

Alford, R. (1975) *Health Care Politics*. University of Chicago Press, Chicago, Illinois.

Basset, G.W. (1971) Change in Australian education. *The Australian Journal of Education*, **15**(1), March.

Benner, P. (1984) *From Novice to Expert*. Addison Wesley, California.

Bennis, W., Benne, K.D. and Chinn, R. (eds) (1988) *The Planning of Change*. Holt, Reinhart and Wilson, New York.

Cantor, M.M. (1973) Philosophy, purpose and objectives; why do we have them? *The Journal of Nursing Administration*, **July–August, 3**(4), 21–25.

Coch, L. and French, J.R.P. (1948) Overcoming resistance to change. Human Relations 1, in *Strategies for Managing Change* (ed W.G. Dyer), Addison Wesley Publishing, New York.

Dalton, G. (1970) Influence and organisational change, in *Organisational Change and Development* (ed L.P. Griener), Irwin Dorsey, Illinois.

Dyer, W.G. (1984) *Strategies for Managing Change*. Addison Wesley Publishing, Reading, Massachusetts.

Evans, K. and Hind, T. (1987) *Nursing Times*, **83**(18).

Fretwell, J.E. (1985) *Freedom to change. The creation of a Ward Learning Environment*. Royal College of Nursing Publications, London.

Gillies, D.A.(1989) *Nursing Management, A systems Approach*, 2nd edn, W.B. Saunders Co/HarcourtBrace Jovanovich Inc., New York.

Giovannetti, P. (1986) Evaluation of primary nursing, in *Annual Review of Nursing Research* (eds H.H. Weilty, J.J. Fitzpatrick and R.L. Taunton), Springer Publishing Co., New York.

Graham, I. (1991) Primary Nursing: Accountability if the Key to its Mystery. *Nursing Practice (Nursing Standard)*, **4**(2).

Cuba, D. and Clark, D.L. (1978) Planned organisational change in education, in *Curriculum Innovation* (eds A. Harris et al.), Croom Helm, London.

Hibbs, P. (1988) *Pressure Area Care for the City and Hackney Health Authority*. City and Hackney Health Authority, West Smithfield, London.

Homans, G.C. (1981) The human group, in *Implementing Change in Nursing* (eds E.G. Mauksch and M.H. Miller), C.V. Mosby Co., London.

Imershein, A. (1977) Organisational change as a paradigm shift. *The Sociological Quarterly*, **Winter, 18**(1), 33–43.

Kings Fund Centre (1986) *Quality Circles.* Kings Fund, London.

Lewin, K. (1953) Studies in group decisions, in *Group Dynamics: Research and Theory* (eds D. Cartwright and A. Zander), Row Peterson, Evanston, Illinois.

Macdonald, M. (1988) Primary nursing; is it worth it? *Journal of Advanced Nursing,* **13**, 797–806.

MacGuire, J. (1989) Primary nursing, a better way to care? *Nursing Times,* **85**(46), 50–3.

Marriner-Tomey, A. (1988) *Guide to Nursing Management,* 3rd edn. Mosby Mission, St. Louis, Louisiana.

Pembrey, S. (1989) The development of nursing practice, a new contradiction. *Senior Nurse,* **9**(8), 3–8.

Pembrey, S. and Punton, S. (1990) The lessons of nursing beds. *Nursing Times,* **86**(14), 44–45.

Plant, R. (1987) *Managing Change and Making it Stick.* Fontana paperbacks, London.

Pratt (1982) in Greaves, F. (1982) Innovation, change, decision making and the key variables in nursing curriculum implementation. *International Journal of Nursing Studies,* **19**(1).

Reed, J.A. (1988) A comparison of nurse related behaviour, philosophy of care and job satisfaction in team and primary nursing. *Journal of Advanced Nursing,* **13**, 383–95.

Rogers (1979) cited in Welch, L.B. (1979) Planned change in nursing. *Nursing Clinics of North America,* **14**(2), 311.

Smith G. and Cantley, C. (1985) *Assessing Health Care. A Study in Organisational Evaluation* . Open University Press, Buckingham.

Stocking, B. (1984) *Initiative of Inertia. Burgess and Son, Oxfordshire.*

Webb, C. (1989) Action Research: Philisophy, methods and personal experience. *Journal of Advanced Nursing,* **14**, 403–410.

5

A systematic approach for changing the way of organizing nursing work in a clinical setting

Chapter 4 introduced an assessment tool that we found useful when planning to change the nursing work methodology in the clinical setting (Table 4.2). Two of the factors identified in the assessment tool have been explored: change management theories and work methodology. The other factors identified were:

- Factor 3 – nursing role.
- Factor 4 – nurse accountability.
- Factor 5 – environment.
- Factor 6 – workload systems.
- Factor 7 – leadership style.
- Factor 8 – communications.
- Factor 9 – quality assurance.

This chapter will explore each of these in more detail, with descriptions of the process of implementing these in a clinical setting, based on our own practical experiences. This will be followed by an overview of how all of these factors can be utilized when developing a strategic plan for the systematic implementation of a new work methodology. The first of these factors pertains to the nursing role.

FACTOR 3: THE NURSING ROLE

'Role' has been defined as 'A pattern of behaviour that characterizes and is expected of a person who occupies a certain position in a group or social organisation' (Raven and Rubin, 1983).

An important consideration is the role of the nurse in relation to the larger structure of the functioning of the hospital, and the different roles of different grades of staff within the nursing hierarchy. Determining the nursing role at macro and micro level is important, as it is only by defining the roles in this way that staff gain a clear indication of the parameters within which they can practice. Therefore the role of the nurse within a given context determines the intellectual and physical work they will actually carry out.

In our assessment tool (Table 4.2) the two ends of the continuum for assessing the nursing role range between a restricted role, with nursing as a practical activity, and with an emphasis on technical skills and, at the other extreme, the expansion of the nursing role, with nursing seen as an intellectual activity and with an emphasis on creativity. It is crucial to make an honest assessment of the current position on the assessment tool for the area targeted for changing the work methodology of the nursing role.

In our experience, failure to move well over to the right of the continuum before implementing the new work methodology, leads to a situation we refer to as 'lip-service Primary Nursing'. These are wards that have all the visible trappings of a trendy, forward thinking, place to work. The photos are on the board, there are lots of glossy leaflets about the place and all patients have a named nurse. Closer examination of the ward routine, however, shows a traditional, task-allocated approach to care delivery. Visible signs that this is occurring include the Sister or Charge Nurse doing all the ward and drug rounds, beds all made before breakfast, all the 'work' (e.g. dressings, specimen collections, etc.) done before the late shift come on, poorly written care plans with no clear patient goals and infrequent evaluations.

In practice, moving staff along the continuum to the stage where they have the competence and confidence to function in this new, expanded role is a time-consuming and challenging process. The degree of personal change it requires in an individual is also stressful and can be very threatening, both for them and for the hierarchy. It requires the managers to take risks and allow the development of new, innovative practices, which means giving up a lot of the 'position power' that comes with a hierarchical post. Having staff question practice that is well established in a manager's area of responsibility can be taken as a personal attack on their professional integrity if the process is not carefully managed.

Similarly, as part of the creative, intellectual process, questioning all aspects of their own nursing practice and using a research-based approach to nursing care can be threatening for staff, who may feel they are being told that what they have done in the past is 'wrong'. This third factor on the assessment tool is therefore closely linked with that of communications (Factor 8) and, in particular, strategies identified as part of this factor, such as team building. It is important to start from the basis of building on the positive aspects of previous practice, and not to devalue staff by appearing overly critical of all aspects of previous approaches.

When examining the factor of the nurse's role in relation to the work methodology, in order to make an accurate assessment, the workload systems explored later in this chapter can be useful in establishing exactly what it is the nurses spend their time doing. A common finding in reviewing the literature concerning the role of the nursing staff and organization of care is that it is often the staff with the least training (often auxiliary nurses) who give the highest proportion of direct care. The trained staff spend more time on administration and assisting the medical staff, believing these to be more prestigious activities (Savage et al., 1979; Wells, 1980). These findings were mirrored in our own areas of practice. If the nurse's role and nursing work are perceived in this way, then it will be extremely difficult to create a dynamic, creative approach to nursing care.

Developing the nursing role is therefore dependent on preparing the nurse for the new responsibility and then creating a work methodology that enables him or her to put the intellectual and creative components of their work into practice. There is little point doing one without the other.

The issues concerned with skill mix and grade mix are reviewed in the section on factor 6 (workload systems). However, once the numbers of staff have been allocated to a ward, the change agent and the staff need to be quite clear in their own minds on the function and purpose of all the roles within the team.

Under a task allocated system, the grade of staff and position they held within the hierarchy of a particular shift would determine the work that a member of staff would carry out. For example, the person in charge would do the doctor's rounds, drug rounds and give reports; the second most senior did the dressings and wrote care plans, with other, 'lower', grades washing patients, giving out bedpans, etc. (Manthey, in Macdonald, 1988). With the exception of the ward Sister or Charge Nurse, or those at the bottom of the pecking order, this meant that the tasks carried out from day-to-day would depend on the relative seniority of the staff on duty. It was our experience that the group of staff who fared particularly badly under this system were the enrolled nurses, who on some occasions would be asked to take charge and, on others, would be at the bottom of the hierarchical pile.

To return to the original definition of 'role' as '. . . focusing on a pattern of task-related behaviour as that which characterizes and is expected of a person who occupies a certain position in a . . . social organization' (Raven and Rubin, 1983) it can be appreciated that, for many staff working in a task allocation system of care delivery, their role could change daily. This can cause problems in maintaining the continuity, both in running the ward, and in patient care, as staff switch rapidly between roles. It also means that the less senior staff only get to function 'in charge' when there is no one more experienced to act as a role model, or to offer support. It also places greater value on certain tasks that are seen as more prestigious, rather than on nursing skills related to patient care.

In our early efforts to examine ways in which we could develop the nursing role, it became frustratingly apparent that there will always be a series of mundane, task-related activities that will fall within the nursing domain. Having accepted this, we explored ways in which we could ensure these were carried out, but in a way that made use of the particular skills of individual staff. It also led to our creating new roles within the team – 'Ward Auxiliary' and 'Ward Co-ordinator' – and re-evaluating some of the more traditional roles. We found that by changing these in various ways, we helped to create the climate we were attempting to establish in order to change the work methodology.

The role of the ward sister in relation to implementation of primary nursing

The role of the Ward Sister or Charge Nurse was subject to great debate, and there was a strong feeling that, as this was the individual with the greatest clinical expertise, it was a poor use of our skills if the traditional role allowed us little time for involvement in direct patient care. The debating process with staff and subsequent solutions were important, as the changes in the role were then owned by staff, and it was not seen as the Charge Nurse ducking out of the perceived responsibilities of the post. We felt that the role should shift to developing staff to their full potential, and this would be achieved by setting objectives with them, based on their own personal needs, and working with them in the clinical setting. It was felt that the Charge Nurse working solely with patients would do little to develop the team, and would, in the long run, prove an ineffective use of this individual. It was a case of 'Look after the staff (development), and caring for patients will look after itself.'

The role of Charge Nurse/Sister was therefore changed to focus on service development. This required a massive learning curve on our part, on areas ranging from interview and appraisal skills, objective planning, teaching, team building, research skills and quality management, to name but a few. Although we eventually adapted to the new role, it was not an easy process, and many of our early attempts at coping were based very much on trial and error; until we found a style of leadership with which we felt comfortable, and which served the purpose of effecting the change. We were also helped by various courses that we identified as appropriate for our personal needs.

With hindsight, it would have been extremely useful to have a role model and mentor to help with this process. Many hospitals have recognized the need for such a role and are introducing posts aimed at assisting with the change process. These are appearing with a variety of titles, such as 'Service Development' and 'Clinical Nurse Adviser'. These posts are arising just as some areas are attempting to break the traditional hierarchical structure, and there have been criticisms that they are:

... another constraint on the growth of nursing ... The plethora of rigid rules, regulations, procedures and practice with a clearly defined hierarchy seen within our hospitals is, in itself, antithetical to growth.   (*Vaughn and Pillmoor, 1989*)

It was our experience that to be charged as the sole agent for introducing change was stressful and led to a feeling of isolation. Change Agents often make changes in the system in spite of it, rather than because of it. As Pembrey (1989) observed from her work:

People will try to undermine them precisely because they threaten established practice which is usually more comfortable and requires lesser effort, or because the innovation threatens individuals' or groups' territory, authority, power status or livelihood. Even when an innovation is widely regarded as better, it can fail to become established through lack of support from key people, and much of the investment is lost.

These new Service Development posts offer the potential to assist those in Charge Nurse positions in making the desired changes, without the threat that a direct line management position can often pose.

The success of such positions in facilitating change will inevitably depend on the skills of the postholder, which will be very different from those required in a line management post. It is our observation that the key difference between these individuals and those in traditional hierarchical positions is that the former need to use their personal power, as opposed to the position power of the line manager's post. They therefore need to draw heavily on the change management theories to develop the service by utilizing the skills and enthusiasm of the staff.

We felt that support from such an individual would have been a valuable resource as we grappled for the first time with the concept of Primary Nursing, standard-setting, quality assurance and audit, as well as with the daily ward management.

In order to make time for these new activities, some of the current work tasks that traditionally fell in our domain had to be released. We went through all the traditional tasks identified in our activity sampling and debated whether the Sister really needed to have sole responsibility for them and, if not, the best way of dealing with them. Tasks falling into the category of offering potential to be delegated elsewhere fell into the following groupings:

- Administrative.
- Co-ordinating the work activity for the shift.
- 'Fire-fighting' and trouble-shooting.
- Tasks that no one could identify a purpose in completing. We resolved them in the following ways.

Delegation of administrative tasks

The administrative element fell into two categories – nursing administration and general administration. For the nursing administration, it was agreed that paperwork arising directly from patients would be dealt with by the team leader (or, later, by the Primary or Associate Nurse) from whose patients it arose (e.g. all care plans and evaluations, incident forms, reports, etc.).

For the general administration, it was agreed to change the role of one of the auxiliaries to include the general administrative duties necessary to run the ward. We called this post the 'Ward Auxiliary'. One area did not have a ward clerk, and a considerable amount of nursing time was spent on these duties. Establishing this role involved setting clear requirements on how these duties should be completed, and an initial period of supervision. The Ward Auxiliary was then able to order all the stores, book all ambulance and outpatient appointments, prepare all paperwork for admission and discharges and perform numerous other activities, including non-administrative work. This included stripping and making beds when patients were discharged, giving out menus and helping patients complete them, checking equipment, completing and chasing works requisition forms, searching for lost items, taking urgent requisitions to the Pharmacy and Pathology Laboratory and collecting discharge medication for patients, general tidying of the ward area, keeping the noticeboard and patient allocation board up to date, escorting non-acute patients to X-ray and offering clerical support to the Charge Nurse and other staff. We found that the expanded role of the Charge Nurse required good secretarial support.

Delegation of co-ordinating the work activity for the shift

The second area that offered the potential to be delegated from the Charge Nurse/Sister role was co-ordinating the work for the shift. This also fell into two categories – co-ordinating patient care and general ward co-ordination.

Co-ordinating patient care
It was agreed that all aspects relating to patient care would be co-ordinated by the nurse looking after the patient. Hence they would go on the ward round for their patients, ensure relevant referrals were made and that discharge planning was completed, etc. It was also agreed they would do all their own drug administration and teaching, and abandon the practice of the person 'in charge' doing all these.

General ward co-ordination
There was also a strong feeling that one individual needed to have an overall picture of what was happening on a ward on each shift. There was a need to make decisions as to which team new admissions should be allocated and generally to co-ordinate the smooth running of the ward to allow the other staff to concentrate solely on patient care. Analysis of the skills required for this role led to the conclusion that this need not be the person most senior in the hierarchy. It was felt that all trained staff could develop through rotating into this role, and that less experienced staff could benefit in trying it when they knew more experienced staff were on duty. The role of 'Ward Co-ordinator' was created to fulfil this function. The nurses responsible for their patients would keep the Co-ordinator informed of all developments related to them. The Co-ordinator for each shift was highlighted on the off-duty, and the role shared out equally between all trained staff. Staff were not given the role after days off, as it was important they had worked at least one shift and knew a fair proportion of the patients. In practice this worked extremely well, and prevented the ludicrous situation of the Sister coming back off annual leave on a Monday morning and attempting to co-ordinate the ward, as well as being expected to answer questions on a ward round concerning patients she had never nursed.

Delegation of fire-fighting and trouble-shooting

The third major area identified as taking up a significant amount of the Sister or Charge Nurses's time was fire-fighting and trouble-shooting. This meant dealing with all the 'gremlins' that crop up routinely, and can take a considerable amount of sorting out, from ambulances not turning up, stock items running out, lack of linen, patient complaints, staff sickness and arranging subsequent cover; the list was endless. Initially our solution was to allocate these to the Ward Co-ordinator or the Ward Auxiliary, depending on the type of problem. Later, as our knowledge of quality improvement increased, it became apparent it would be far more effective to be proactive, and stop the problems from arising in the first place. This was the final piece in the jigsaw of our quest for managing quality, and is covered in detail in Chapter 6.

Delegation of tasks that no one could identify a purpose in completing

The final group of tasks we came across were those that we had carried out unquestioningly since the dawn of time and which, on reflection, served no useful purpose. A good place to start is a review of paperwork. On chasing up all the routine forms we were expected to complete, it was interesting to be told by one recipient 'We don't really know what to do with them, we just file them'. Another area worth examining is attendance at meetings. This is covered in more detail in Chapter 6, but often we found we were invited to meetings at which our attendance served no useful purpose, either in helping fulfil the objective of the meeting, or to ourselves. The traditional style 'unit meeting' was another example, which consisted mainly of information-giving, based on memorandums that had already been circulated to the wards. A final note; if (as many of our activity sampling exercises indicated) any nursing time is spent on 'weekend cleaning', we suggest that immediate attention be given to this (worryingly common) activity. In our experience, a significant proportion of the most senior staff on the ward (whilst paid time and two-thirds on a Sunday) were spending their time cleaning out cupboards and defrosting drug fridges, amongst other domestic tasks.

Solutions included delegation of tasks to a more appropriate member of staff, rescheduling the routine weekly cleaning when staff were not on unsocial hours rates and ensuring that senior staff were rostered on duty when their skills were most needed.

The above strategies and actions enabled us to establish a system that offered the trained staff on the ward a role model and experienced senior member of staff who now had the time to dedicate to their professional development. It also relieved trained staff of the majority of the non-nursing duties that had previously reduced the amount of time they were able to spend in direct patient care. This had begun to move us along the continuum for factor 3 on our assessment tool (Table 4.2), towards developing the intellectual and creative aspects of the nursing role.

Many of the strategies outlined above were formulated during the 'time out' from the ward dedicated to team building. It was in these sessions that staff raised issues that were of concern to them relating to the change towards Primary Nursing. When considering this Factor, two major concerns relating to the development of the intellectual and creative aspects of their role in relation to preparing for the new system were given priority for action. These were: (i) the advanced clinical and theoretical knowledge; and (ii) advanced inter-personal skills that were felt to be necessary. Strategies used for developing these components are outlined below.

Strategies for developing advanced clinical and theoretical skills and knowledge

We identified that, with the increased autonomy and account-ability that accompanied the new approach, many staff were concerned that their traditional training and subsequent paucity of post-basic development had not prepared them adequately with sufficiently advanced clinical or theoretical knowledge to function confidently in the new roles of Primary or Associate Nurse under the new system.

When discussing the development of clinical knowledge, it was felt that it was unrealistic to expect each member of staff to be an 'expert' in everything. The team brainstormed areas in which they felt increased knowledge to enable them to care for the sorts of nursing problems that were typically representative in patients admitted to the ward was needed, and came up with the following list:

- Wound care.
- Pressure sore prevention and management.
- Continence management.
- Management of diabetes.
- Managing patients with acute myocardial infarction, including interpretation of ECGs.
- Infection control.
- Rehabilitation.
- Nursing models, nursing care plans and nursing theory.
- Research techniques.
- Management of patients with breathlessness.
- Health promotion.
- Management of patients with pain.
- Nursing patients with differing religious beliefs.
- Standard setting.
- Legal and ethical issues.
- Complementary therapies.
- Rest and sleep.

Each member of staff then selected one of the above that they wished to take responsibility for.

All staff were seen on an individual basis to discuss professional development and jointly agreed objectives; target dates for completed actions were set. We found it useful to review these three times a year. The objectives included developing their knowledge on the selected topic chosen, and establishing ways of sharing this with the rest of the team. Methods staff selected for disseminating knowledge included teaching sessions, preparing resource packs, preparing a poster display for the noticeboard, practical demonstrations, developing audit tools and inviting outside speakers into the hospital.

The latter approach was particularly useful for formulating our aims and objectives related to discharge and rehabilitation planning. We were fortunate in gaining the co-operation of former patients with disabilities, who came to talk openly to us about their experience in hospital. Hearing from a profoundly visually handicapped gentleman how he was regularly told in one outpatient department to 'find a seat'; how the domestic left a bucket of water by his bed, which he put his foot in; how staff persisted in cutting all his food into tiny pieces; how staff walked off without telling him they were leaving, leaving him talking to thin air; how he pulled down his pyjamas in the expectation of an injection not realizing the nurse was talking to (and pulling the curtain around) the patient in the next bed, was a humbling and deeply insightful experience for all of us. Listening to these, and other accounts, we realized it was not enough to concentrate just on developing the trained staff, and where it was appropriate, untrained staff were also included in educational sessions.

Staff were helped to develop their knowledge in the selected area of interest by being funded to go on related study days and conferences, allowed time to study in the library, and by having short clinical attachments with individuals who already had specialist knowledge. In topics which were predominantly related to a medical condition, the staff were encouraged to forge strong links with the consultant medical staff with special interest in this area, both for support, and to prevent potential conflicts of interest arising. In practice, some extremely fruitful working relationships developed, and the medical staff proved useful allies in removing potential road blocks to progress.

We found this approach as useful, as all staff help to develop the knowledge of the others, whilst developing themselves professionally and gaining skills in teaching, and other methods of presentation. It also meant that there was a pool of specialist knowledge within the team that all could utilize. For example, the nurse caring for a patient with a problematic wound could refer to the individual with expertise in this area for advice. It also incorporates many of the key approaches advocated in the theories of managing change, such as ownership and encouraging a free exchange of ideas to develop participation, as well as offering the potential for job enrichment; a factor identified as important in motivating staff (Hertzberg, 1968).

The presence of an individual with an interest in care planning and nursing thoery was also found to be advantageous. Our original care plan audit showed the need for improvement in this area. There was little point in developing all the other areas if nothing was ever documented properly to allow evaluation and continuity of care, notwithstanding the legal implications relating to poor documentation.

Having identified and implemented our strategies for

improving the theoretical and clinical knowledge of staff in preparation for their new role as Primary or Associate Nurses, the second issue necessary for moving this factor along the continuum towards the nursing role being a creative and intellectual activity was explored.

Strategies used for developing interpersonal skills and knowledge

The second area that was highlighted by staff as needing further development for their new role was improving interpersonal skills. We identified that a major source of stress in our work was in handling conflict situations, either with patients, relatives or staff; or in telling people things we knew they would find distressing. After considerable discussion, the team identified the following areas as priorities for action:

- Counselling skills.
- Dealing with bereavement.
- Communication skills (including telephone skills).
- Assertiveness skills.
- Stress management and relaxation.
- Team building.

Some of the methods useful in developing these skills are outlined elsewhere (Evans and Hind, 1987; Evans and Slater, 1990; Slater, 1990). We recommend the use of skilled facilitators to run these courses as, badly handled, they can provide a potential source of conflict which is counterproductive to their aim. We were fortunate in identifying local staff with these skills, which made the sessions very cost-effective. We have found the health promotion and personnel departments useful sources of staff with such skills. These individuals organized workshops on the above themes to meet our objectives (Evans and Hind, 1987).

These strategies helped us to overcome two potential restraining forces to implementing the new work methodology, namely insufficient advanced clinical and theoretical knowledge, and lack of confidence by individuals in their interpersonal skills in the areas listed above, and prepared staff for their new role.

At this point in the change process, when staff felt confident that they were ready to take on the new system for organizing nursing work, a consensus on the form this should take was needed.

We would reiterate our earlier advice that team nursing is a good starting point to wean staff in gently to the new way of working. It enables the team leader to get used to the responsibility of caring for a caseload of patients, and functioning in a more autonomous role. Later, one needs to decide who will be Primary and who Associate Nurses. (The role of the Associate Nurse is to carry out the prescribed nursing care as directed by the Primary Nurse.)

Selecting staff for the role of Primary or Associate Nurse

There are no clear-cut answers as to who should be the Primary and who the Associate Nurse, they need to be resolved at a local level. Considerations need to be given to the following issues:

- *Qualifications and experience.* In our experience, our selection criteria stated that the nurse should be qualified for a minimum of 1 year before being considered for this role. This was to allow them time to develop their knowledge and gain experience under the guidance of a Primary Nurse after graduation.
- *Settling-in period.* We also found it important to give all new nurses a settling-in period of 3 months as an Associate Nurse before deciding whether they wished to be considered for the role of Primary Nurse.
- *Team leader abilities.* All staff coped well in fulfilling the role of Team Leader for the shift.
- *Previous experience.* This was another criterion for consideration.

A factor that will influence this decision is the skill mix on the ward at the time. There is a continuous debate as to whether or not enrolled nurses should function in the role of Primary Nurse or Team Leader, with some areas changing their skill mix as part of the change process (Binnie, 1987).

In our location, changing the skill mix to one of predominantly Registered Nurses was not an option available to us and, unless some Enrolled Nurses had agreed to accept the role, we could not have progressed any further with the changes. In practice, these individuals coped well with the challenge, and gave up a considerable amount of their own time to attend courses to help develop skills and knowledge needed for the role. We would not advocate that all Enrolled Nurses could adequately fulfil the role of Primary Nurse, but the fact that some Registered Nurses were unable to cope with this responsibility highlighted the need to base the decision on individual competence and performance; and for the decision to be made in conjunction with the member of staff concerned.

The Nursing Role in a wider context

Having developed the nursing role within the ward team at a micro level, it is advantageous to consider the nursing role within the social organization of the hospital, and also the broader political context. A large part of highlighting the role of the nurse is reliant on establishing communication links with other professionals and departments.

Initially, we were very good at complaining amongst ourselves about what we perceived as a lack of power of the nursing profession influencing corporate decision making, as opposed to that of other groups within the organization within the hospital. We were also very bad at doing anything to strengthen the nursing role at this level, and tended to be reactive, rather than proactive, in our approach.

Strategies to strengthen our role and raise the profile of professional nursing within the organization

First, we considered our public relations strategy. We identified key individuals within the organization who we had never met. We then invited them for an informal meeting with staff to enable us to introduce ourselves and hear about their role, and explain ours. All invited personnel came.

We then worked towards fostering these professional relationships to mutual advantage, as outlined at the end of this section.

Once links had been established with other areas of the hospital, the next aim was to raise the profile of the nursing profession within it. Techniques used to achieve this are outlined under Factor 8 (Communication).

We made a conscious effort to attend the organizational meetings that we had previously avoided, and to contribute actively to these. Volunteering for local committees and project groups proved another successful strategy in gaining input to local decision making.

On an even broader level, the need to raise the profile and status of the role of nursing in society was acknowledged as important. This can be partially addressed by taking a more politically active role; working with community and organizational groups outside the hospital, and use of the media.

The above strategies were all instrumental in helping us to move the third factor identified on our assessment tool along the continuum in preparation for Primary Nursing by expanding our role. As our knowledge-base increased; so too did our understanding of some of the more subtle implications of implementing a new work methodology. One of these was the close interrelationship between our expanding role as practitioners and our professional accountability. This is the fourth factor in our assessment tool (Table 4.2) and will now be explored.

FACTOR 4: NURSE ACCOUNTABILITY

Accountability has been defined as: '. . . being responsible for one's acts and being able to define or measure in some way the results of the decision making.'

The United Kingdom Central Council (UKCC) code of professional conduct states that nurses are primarily accountable to patients (UKCC, 1984). Exercising accountability involves the nurse using his or her professional judgement and being answerable for that judgement, being accountable not only for acts, but also for omissions. It was envisaged that the UKCC code of conduct would therefore place the power and duty to exercise accountability with individual practitioners.

In practice, we identified the necessity to move along the continuum outlined in our assessment tool (Table 4.2) from one where accountability is diffuse, with deference to medicine, to the nurse being accountable and autonomous for his or her practice (Manthey, 1980).

Of all the identified factors, this was the one that caused staff the most concern. Many felt that it left them personally very vulnerable, and felt extremely threatened at the potential consequences.

Even the role of 'Team Leader' led to reservations from some staff. Moving from a culture where most actions were invariably sanctioned by the person in charge, to one that places the decision making with the practitioner proved to be a difficult and time-consuming process, which, for reasons outlined below, we were unable to complete fully, and could not move to the far right of our assessment tool.

An early miscalculation during our assessment phase was to under-estimate just how ingrained in the nursing culture was the habit of referring all decisions 'up the line'. We found numerous examples where the traditional hierarchical structure re-inforced the dependence of all grades of staff on others in making decisions for them by creating a set of rules and regulations to maintain the hierarchical status quo. There were examples of Senior Sisters and Charge Nurses needing to ring the Clinical Manager for 'permission' to book a hospital taxi for transfer of urgent specimens, a rule to go through the Senior Nurse on duty to get 'permission' to borrow linen from the reserve store and the need to have all stock requisitions checked and countersigned; the list was endless. The most ludicrous of all such examples was on the rare occasions we actually experienced a spell of hot weather, we all had to wait expectantly for the letter of special dispensation to arrive, giving us 'permission' to take our tights off! It was against a backdrop of such an organizational culture (that created for many staff the impression they were unable to be trusted with making the most trivial decisions) that we were talking about autonomy and accountability.

The disparity was made obvious when, in an inaugural ward meeting, on asking the staff's opinion on something, there was a stunned silence. After a few moments, one of them put their hand up, which (we learned later) was for permission to speak! Within such a climate there is a need for an enormous amount of preparatory work encompassed in the other factors on our assessment tool before the nursing role can expand to anything approaching an autonomous and accountable practitioner.

We use the word 'approaching', but we found, in practice, that this factor proved extremely difficult to move along the continuum on our assessment tool. First, from a professional perspective, even at Sister grade we had very limited control over our work situation. We had no budget or financial control, no input into determining our staff establishment figures, limited input into strategic planning and many of us were labouring in wards designed a century ago and which were now completely unsuited for their current use. Hence the importance of the environmental factor and that of workload dependency, both of which can have a profound impact on nurse accountability, demonstrating the interdependence on all of these when managing the change to Primary nursing.

Under these theses circumstances, the fairness of demanding accountability from someone for aspects of nursing care that may be affected by factors that are outside their control is questionable. This was noted in another study, which found that the ward sister had much responsibility, but little autonomy and authority (Pembrey, 1978).

There is also the potential for nurse accountability to conflict directly with the medical profession. In the UK, as the law stands at the moment, the current Doctor/Nurse relationship limits the extent to which the nurse can claim primacy.

Despite these difficulties, we identified a number of strategies to help move this factor from left to right along the continuum on our assessment tool. These are outlined below.

Strategies for developing nurse accountability and autonomy

One strategy that helped us move towards a heightened awareness of our accountability and explore the concept of autonomy was in having the team member responsible for legal and ethical issues research these areas and prepare a resource pack for the team.

A number of staff attended study days on these themes and issues identified on these days were raised at ward level to discuss local implications and actions.

Another issue relating to accountability that required clarification with management was the whole area of vicarious liability, particularly in relation to nurses taking on extended roles which may necessitate staff to complete further training and certification if the nurse is to be protected in this way by the employer. The introduction of the 'scope of professional practice' (UKCC, 1992) poses further challenges for the nursing role.

In spite of some difficulties, we found the process of moving partway along the continuum towards accountability and autonomy a worthwhile one. One of the most beneficial aspects of considering these concepts was it began to change our attitude towards the role of the traditionally passive, accepting role of the nurse, to the recognition that we were required to justify our rationale for the care we gave. Many staff had been ignorant of the implications of the UKCC code of conduct, and were labouring under the misapprehension that if things went wrong it was the nurse in charge who would 'carry the can'. It also helped to introduce patients' rights and ethical issues into the planning meetings, which led to many of us developing our thoughts and attitudes on aspects of care we had not previously debated as a team. We also felt a moral obligation that staff should be fully aware of the implications the expanded role and changing work methodology would place upon them.

It was during these discussions that two items appeared regularly on the agenda. The first was the restraints placed on developing the role of the nurse and being accountable and autonomous by what we termed loosely 'environmental factors'. The second was the restraints that arose because of the current skill mix of staff. These two factors, and the impact they had on our attempts to change the work methodology are outlined below.

FACTOR 5: ENVIRONMENT

One of the restraining forces we identified in implementing the change to the new work methodology, was that we often become oblivious to many of the detrimental factors that were affecting the quality of service in our ward. Those relating to attitudes and behaviour have already been addressed through other factors on the assessment scale. Those relating to the environment were similarly difficult to objectively define.

The following methods were found useful in helping us to define these environmental factors:

- At the start of the change process, invite an objective outside observer to come to the hospital, find their way to the ward, sit on it for an hour and write down their experiences and impressions.

- Ask staff to brainstorm all the things to do with the physical environment that would create an unfavourable impression if they were a patient. Use this information as a central focus when designing the ward philosophy.

We were keen that what was written in the philosophy, and the plans of care that we were prescribing for our patients should be an accurate reflection of what happened in practice. On closer scrutiny, many of the typical statements commonly found in these documents began to resemble jargon from an estate agent's brochure. We offer the following glossary of terms, based on many of the difficulties we have experienced in correlating the quality statements offered, with the standard of service given.

Glossary of typical quality statements

Respect dignity and privacy

There will be 6 feet between your bed and that of neighbouring other patients. Curtains will be pulled round for privacy, but they will be too short and you will be aware of a gap through which you are convinced that the man in the opposite bed is watching the Doctor give you a pelvic floor examination. Fellow patients hear a full account of the medical history you give to the Doctor, and you will have your bowels opened in full hearing of the patient in the next bed. Hospital nightwear can be provided, following the top selling design of the 'buttock-exposer' theatre wear, which is modelled by other patients coming back from their pre-operative shower. Bathroom doors never seem to have locks that work, and in case you find one that does, your moment of solitude is broken by a nurse with a special key to get in. Whilst the nurse is helping you to bathe, colleagues will continually throw the door open and enquire cheerily 'Have you got the drug keys?'

Provide individualized care based on patients' personal needs

You will report to the ward at 8 a.m. on Monday morning with eight other patients for admission. The ward is very efficient,

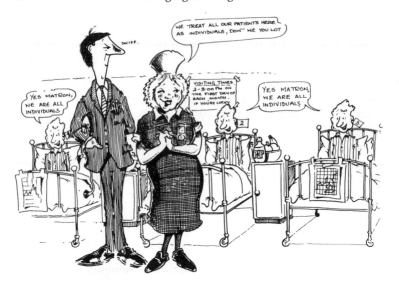

Illustration 5.1 Individualized care.

and all the beds are named and care plans already written. You have difficulty walking, but even the bed closest to the toilet is a considerable distance. There is nowhere in the ward where you can phone your family. The ward lights are switched off at 10 p.m. and on at 7 a.m. The chairs are too low for you to get out of and the bed tables are so high that if you have to eat in bed you need a set of crampons to reach the plate. The toilet rolls are in a big plastic dispenser and you need a degree to work out how to get any paper out. You also need flexible fingers and good eyesight and co-ordination to manoeuvre it through the 1 cm serrated plastic edge which dispenses one piece of toilet paper at a time. The television is left on all day. The ward is short of wash bowls, so you share one with your neighbour. If you are wheelchair-bound, the sinks are all too high for you to wash yourself. If you are partially sighted, the 'clutter' around the ward makes it difficult for you to get around safely. There is a handwritten notice stating the visiting times, and banning children under eight from entering the ward.

Treat all individuals equally, and with respect regardless of sex, race, colour or creed

The menu offers fish and chips or roast beef and Yorkshire pudding. There is a bible in your locker. All the hospital notices and a lot of the written information is in English. Female nursing staff are not allowed to wear trousers and must wear hats. The medical staff eat in a separate dining room.

Our aim is to provide a high standard of service

The sheets on your bed will have suspicious looking stains. The radio headset by your bed is broken and the fluorescent light flickers constantly. The bathroom is cold and bare, and hasn't been painted for 10 years. The wheelchair used to take you to X-ray has no footrests and you have to be wheeled through the hospital holding your legs in the air to prevent certain amputation. The meals are cold and not what you ordered. You ask for something to read and are given a 1978 copy of *The Peoples' Friend*. You seem to have to wait for long periods of time in all departments before being seen and it takes you ages to find them because they are so poorly signposted. There is no chair by your bed. The nightwear is patched and worn and all the buttons are missing. Your bed is at a fixed height and you are unable to climb into it.

Create a quiet, relaxing environment to alleviate stress and promote sleep

You will sleep in a room with 28 other people, and the one in the next bed snores loudly in between shouting 'The Doctors are coming!' There are no night lights and the main corridor lights are left on. The plumbing rattles and shakes all night and a tap dancing elephant keeps shining a torch in your face. A telephone rings continuously and patient call bells are loud enough to be measured on the Richter scale.

Staff health and safety is our priority

Female staff will be provided with a uniform that makes it impossible to lift properly without being arrested for indecent exposure. The circa 1948 lifting aid with threadbare calico hoist has been awaiting repair for months. The lack of space between beds makes it impossible to get into all those marvellous lifting positions demonstrated by the physiotherapist. The central stores persistently runs out of disposable gloves. The security officer retired from the fire service on grounds of ill health 15 years ago and is of limited use when patients become violent. The nurses are forbidden to use the car park closest to the wards (which is kept for administrative staff) necessitating a long walk to an unlit carpark late at night.

We will encourage the professional development of all our staff

The nurse training budget for the whole hospital is £2000. Management have frozen all study leave until the current financial overspend has been resolved.

Although 'tongue in cheek', this glossary illustrates the enormous restrictions that the environment places on being able to translate those well-meaning words into a reality. In practice, this makes staff and patients very cynical about philosophical and value statements. If the philosophy and prescribed care are to be taken seriously, these environmental issues must be addressed, and resolved, in order to support changes in the other factors identified.

In our assessment tool, the minimum position on the continuum for this factor shows the nurses having little devolution of responsibility, and little control of their environment. In our experience, nurses at ward level were seldom consulted or given the opportunity to contribute to decisions taken regarding their working environment. Planning teams came and went, building strategies were devised and, at the end of it all, we were stuck with what we were given. The stream of resulting anecdotes is endless; the new gastroscopy suite with doors too narrow to get the beds in; the new X-ray equipment that was too tall for the room it was to go in, requiring the floor to be dug out; the new portacabin, which when lowered by a crane onto its base was too near to a wall to open the doors; the long-awaited new bath being plumbed in flush to the wall, making it impossible to get a hoist round it; the sinks aimed at being the right height for wheelchair users having a vanity unit built round them, which unfortunately prevented wheelchairs getting in close enough to use the sink.

The other big restraining force on us being able to have any input into our environment was lack of money. We did not hold the budget for equipment or maintenance, and were therefore reliant on those who did to provide for us.

But perhaps the saddest aspect of the above scenario was that the nursing staff had resigned themselves to the fact that all of this was inevitable, and did not perceive it as part of the nursing role to become involved in environmental planning or maintenance. This is in spite of the correlation between environment and health. In the long run, working in a dingy ward with poor equipment is as frustrating and morale sapping for staff as patients. Even the best intentioned primary nurse cannot give prescribed care with limited resources and equipment.

It is therefore important to move along the continuum to the other extreme, where there is much devolution of responsibility, allowing staff to control their environment. The following approaches are recommended, as they were instrumental in helping us to achieve this:

Strategies for moving along the change continuum for Factor 5 (environment)

Our first strategy involved finding out which individuals were responsible for different environmental factors as, in practice, budgets seemed to be split between different individuals in a number of different ways.

We established good networks of communication with these individuals and found out what their plans and priorities were. The next stage was to raise their awareness of the current problems, in a way that did not cause them to feel threatened, criticized or defensive. Our interpersonal skills training proved useful for this purpose.

In many instances, it was our own fault these difficulties had continued, as we had often never let these individuals know there was a problem.

A useful approach is to negotiate the establishment of a multidisciplinary task group, to explore ways for improving the ward environment. Budget holders, interested professionals and any other individuals known of locally who will be an asset to the group can be invited to join, explaining what their purpose in the group would be. This should include those with special skills (we recommend the hospital gardener, artistic staff, etc.), local fund-raising groups, the health and safety representative and, of course, nursing staff. Using the 'corrective action team' approach, and some of the 'quality circle' techniques, current problems can be identified and resolved by this group, and future improvements planned. It is important that this task force includes members who have the power and authority to act outside the meeting, and to focus on actions as well as creative ideas.

Such a forum is an excellent venue for facilitating nursing input at more senior levels, allowing them increased control over the ward environment. Our rationale for attempting such an approach was heavily influenced by Kanter's (1983) three methods for improving power access: (i) open communication systems; (ii) network-forming devices (which help to create coalitions of supporters); and (iii) decentralization of resources.

Having gained managerial support, and this being clearly demonstrated to staff by the nature of the improvements made by the group, the next stage is to empower the staff to make their own inputs into improving their work environment.

An extremely effective way of doing this in our early stages of change, was by the use of 'personalizing the service' workshops, started as an initiative by Trent Regional Health Authority (Liddle and Kaye, 1991). These comprised a half-day introductory session and a 1- or 2-day workshop. The content comprised an introduction by a member of senior management, confirming their commitment to the initiative and their views on its benefits. This was followed by ice-breaking exercises, general introductions and a video outlining projects completed by previous participants. An ex-patient with previous admissions in a number of UK hospitals presented a 'patient's-eye view' of some of his interesting, and not always pleasant, hospital experiences. This formed the basis for debate and opened the floor for the rest of the days, in which staff were required to develop an action plan for a project aimed at promoting a more personal service for patients, using their peers to build on and assist with their ideas. A follow-up session was held 6 months later, where staff prepared poster presentations on the impact of their project, and the resultant exhibition was open to the senior managers, hospital staff, public and the local press.

The staff involved in this initiative proved to be extremely creative and demonstrated great pride in their work. The exhibition was a way for managers and peers to recognize their achievement. One benefit was in the large numbers of projects, which led to a demonstrable improvement in the environment. These staff achieved goals in a way no one individual in charge of a ward could have achieved in years; and these projects were completed in 6 months.

Examples include the establishment of a children's play area on a male surgical ward for the large numbers of visiting children; the transformation of a junk room into a wallpapered, carpeted 'quiet room' for use by bereaved relatives; another dingy room redecorated and refurbished to allow patients and relatives to spend time together away from the ward; yet another disused room refurbished and redecorated to provide a private area for admission interviews to take place; the purchase of a tea trolley with china cups and saucers to provide patients using an oncology clinic with refreshment; buying tablecloths and napkins for use on a care of the elderly ward; purchasing duvets with attractive covers; creating a patio garden; buying new curtaining material for the whole hospital; improving entrance areas and improving signposting. Some of these schemes required capital expenditure, which these staff managed to secure from a variety of creative sources. Some of these staff were nurses, but many were auxiliaries, general office staff, porters, sewing room staff, kitchen staff, in fact, anyone who wished to participate.

The initiative caused us to appreciate the extent of the previously untapped resource of staff enthusiasm available when encouraged and facilitated in this way. Used well, it was our most valuable resource.

There were problems with this initiative. Some middle managers felt this approach undermined their authority, and some projects floundered as staff became disillusioned by lack of support.

The final stage was establishing the culture change to enable all staff to contribute in this way to improving the quality of their work.

INTERMEDIATE SUMMARY

A number of factors that are instrumental in the implementation of Primary Nursing into the clinical setting have been identified. In the assessment model (illustrated in Table 4.2) each of these factors is shown along a continuum, and need to be moved from left to right along that continuum to prepare a climate which is conducive to the philosophy of Primary Nursing. The Factors identified are:

- Factor 1 – change management theory.
- Factor 2 – work methodology.
- Factor 3 – nursing role.
- Factor 4 – nurse accountability.
- Factor 5 – environment.
- Factor 6 – workload systems.
- Factor 7 – leadership style.
- Factor 8 – communications.
- Factor 9 – quality assurance.

The first five of these factors have been discussed, with suggested strategies for moving them along to the right hand side of the continuum in Table 4.2. Factor 9 (quality assurance) was discussed in Chapter 3. The remaining three factors that also need to be addressed when planning the change to Primary Nursing will now be explored. The final section in this chapter examines how to develop an implementation strategy that incorporates all of these factors, with consideration for the inter-relationships that exist between them.

FACTOR 6: WORKLOAD SYSTEMS

In attempting to create a climate suitable for changing the work methodology towards one of Primary Nursing, we knew intuitively that the numbers of staff, the grades of staff and the skills of these individuals would be influential to how far we would be able to proceed with its implementation.

There was evidence to suggest that some changes in the skill mix might be necessary to support the new system of working (Binnie, 1987). As part of our strategy for factor 2 (work methodology), we undertook a radical review of the off-duty rota. In examining ways to establish team nursing, we identified that there were insufficient staff of appropriate grades to organize into teams. There was a general expression of concern by staff that they felt the ward to be understaffed for the number of patients. Many pointed out that two new Consultant staff appointments had created an influx of more acutely ill patients, which had further increased the workload on existing staff.

We approached the management and informed them of our need for more staff; we were asked to prove it.

Unfortunately, our arguments were based on subjective feelings, rather than objective facts. It became apparent to us that, in a time of financial restraint, we were going to have to come up with a better argument.

On questioning how the current skill mix had been arrived at, answers were vague, and seemed based on historical tradition. Hence if the ward had always had two sisters, six staff nurses, four enrolled nurses and eight auxiliaries, this is the way things had remained. We reasoned that the ward had become busier; the patients more acute and therefore the staff numbers and skill mix were no longer appropriate; proving this was much more difficult.

As we started to investigate staffing levels, we found that we were also extremely ignorant about how the staff were occupying their time. We needed facts, figures and an objective argument. We needed a workload dependency system.

Introduction to workload dependency systems

There are a number of such systems available on the commercial market. All are aimed at calculating the numbers of staff required to meet the workload of the ward. A summary of the most commonly used approaches we encountered is shown in Table 5.1. There are two commonly used approaches for attempting to develop such systems:

- Those using dependency groupings (or categories).
- Those that assess the number of nursing hours patients require on the basis of task-related interventions, all of which will have been timed previously.

Those using categories (Macintosh, 1987) and criteria (Goldstone et al., 1984) divide patients into a number of groupings with the aim of establishing the average amount of nursing care each

Table 5.1 Model for leading the move towards Primary Nursing

System	Source	Summary
Manchester	MacIntosh (1987)	Based on five dependency categories Workload assessed on nurse time needed per category. Activity sampling carried out
Criteria for care	Goldstone et al. (1984)	Based on four dependency categories Activity sampling carried out. Average timings for set activities
GRASP	Meyer	Assesses number of hours of nursing care each patient will need each day from the nurse care plan
Cheltenham	Bloore (1984)	Based on similar concept to GRASP Activities divided into basic, technical, administrative, domestic and miscellaneous
Rhys Hearn	Rhys Hearn (1974)	Analyses nursing care into 'direct, routine and indirect' care. Indirect and routine care are calculated using bed occupancy Patients are categorized into five groups for basic care and technical care
Aberdeen formula	Stephens et al. (1978)	Patients defined into five care groups and weighting factors determined for each care group based on total amount of care delivered

grouping is likely to require. Initial data collection is therefore required to establish average lengths of nursing time required for all the groupings.

This information can then be used retrospectively or prospectively to predict the amount of staff required on a shift by calculating the number of patients on a ward in each category and multiplying this by the number of nursing hours previously calculated as being required for each category. These systems offer computer software packages to help collate the data.

Utilizing a workload system based on dependency groupings in a clinical setting

When using the Manchester system (Macintosh, 1987) the initial data collection was carried out in two phases. Phase 1 involved activity analysis of the types of activities ward staff carried out for the duration of the shift, including those not relating to direct patient care. Phase 2 involved data collection of a representative sample of five dependency categories, to establish average lengths of nursing time needed for each category. All these data were processed by the software package.

After the data collection and analysis, the wards could report the number of patients in each category and the number of staff hours rostered for the shift; and the software program would indicate whether the rostered staff hours matched the workload. Unlike other systems, this one used the ward staff themselves to collect the data, rather than trained observers. (An example of such data was shown in Figure 4.4.)

Advantages and disadvantages in using either ward staff or external observers for data collection

There were advantages and disadvantages for each of these approaches. In practice, we identified the following difficulties.

In relying on the ward staff to complete their own activity sampling cards, and to record all care given to patients included in the sampling, one makes the assumption that all nurses will fill out the forms honestly and accurately. This was not always the case, and led to two extremes; the example of the night nurse who managed to give patients 15 hours of care on a 10-hour shift; and the example of a category 5 (the highest dependency) patient who, according to the chart, received 3 minutes of nursing care in a 24-hour period.

In relying on trained observers to collect data, there is inevitably the danger of staff being influenced by their presence and changing their normal patterns of working, making the baseline data inaccurate.

Problems found when attempting to identify dependency groupings

Difficulties were experienced when determining the criteria for each of the dependency groupings. The assumption is made in such systems that the low dependency grouping (i.e. virtually self-caring) need proportionately less time than the high dependency groups (i.e. totally dependent on nurses for carrying out most of the activities of daily living).

In practice, we found the dividing line between categories very thin, with many instances of some of the middle categories requiring more time. This was because the totally dependent patients tended to have regular short blocks of care (for example, hourly observations and 2-hourly pressure area care) whereas conscious patients may require more psychological care, taking longer blocks of time (for example, a newly diagnosed insulin-dependent diabetic).

Another concern with this approach of labelling patients within a category was that it created a conflict with our nursing philosophy, which is based on holistic, individualized care. This reductionalist approach of categorizing patients according to the mainly physical tasks that would be done 'for' them seemed to us to be a retrograde step.

We were also concerned that, by focusing on the easily observable, task-related interactions and omitting some of the more sophisticated and less easily measurable interventions (such as assessment and counselling, which often occur simultaneously) a large proportion of work we regarded as the essence of nursing was never accounted for. As Benner (1984) writes 'A sentence cannot be understood by analysing the words alone.'

There was a danger that non-nurses examining such data would assume that 'nursing' involved the list of tasks identified within the categories. In times of financial restraint, this might prove detrimental if a view was formed that such tasks could be carried out by non-trained personnel. There was the possibility that, by following these workload systems without question, the difficulties cited by Smith (1988) might arise namely:

The first step is to measure whatever can be easily measured.
This is OK as far as it goes.
The second step is to disregard that which can't be measured or give it an arbitrary quantitative value.
This is artificial and misleading.
The third step is to presume that what can't be measured easily isn't very important.
This is blindness.
The fourth step is to say that what can't be easily measured really doesn't exist.
This is suicide.

This criticism can also be extended to the other type of dependency tools, which uses activity timings for the most frequently identified nursing activities, which were predominantly task-related (e.g. GRASP). The nurse care plan can then be used to identify which of these activities will be required for each patient for the shift, and it is these that are multiplied to give the total number of nursing hours required.

Another problem found with both types of workload systems is that all data are collected on the assumption that the staffing levels and quality of care on the ward is at an optimum, which may not be the case. For example, using either system, a bed-bath may be identified as taking 10 minutes. This may be because the ward is short staffed and it should actually take 20 minutes to complete properly, or because staff are slower than necessary because they have forgotten half the equipment and keep interrupting the procedure to collect it. Neither does it examine whether the patient actually needed the bed-bath, or the standard of the work carried out.

The link between workload dependency, quality assurance and the nursing role in this example emphasizes the close relationship the nine factors in the assessment tool have in linking together to influence change in the work methodology.

We strongly recommend that a workload dependency system should only be introduced once some form of baseline quality audit has been carried out, hence the importance of the quality assurance factor. Basing staffing levels purely on the workload system in the light of these weaknesses could prove extremely detrimental.

Another factor that influenced the accuracy and subsequent use of the workload system was Factor 1 (change management). In our experience, if staff understood, owned, and could see a WIIFM in any system, the subsequent data would be accurate, and would be used by the staff to help form the basis of action plans for areas highlighted for improvement.

For example, the activity sampling in one area showed a large amount of nurse time spent on non-nursing duties (including weekend cleaning). This highlighted the need for many staff to look at more appropriate ways of delegating these duties. Conversely, in another area, where the workload system was power coercively introduced, little benefit came from the system, which was viewed by staff with hostility as an unnecessary paper exercise.

For this reason, the two ends of the continuum in the assessment tool in Table 4.2 range from a 'top down' implementation and control to one with a 'bottom up' approach that involves staff in its implementation and encourages 'ownership' of it.

Benefits of a workload dependency system when preparing for Primary Nursing

The use of a workload dependency system offered, for the first time, hard data with which management could be approached to demonstrate persistent under-staffing. It also provided us with a method to plot workload trends and plan off-duty more effectively. It was also a useful starting point to explore the area of skill mix.

We identified that it was not just the numbers of staff on a ward that would affect the quality of nursing care given, but the skills of these individuals. Skill mix and grade mix were phrases often used interchangeably, yet the terms are not synonymous. There are many examples of individuals on lower grades who may function at the 'expert' level as defined by Benner (1984). Conversely, there may be those on higher grades who do not possess the same skills. The clinical grading was an attempt to resolve this, although it is debatable to what extent it actually succeeded.

Unfortunately many of the 'job descriptions' for the new grades focus on task- rather than skill-related activities.

Reviewing skill mix prior to the implementation of Primary Nursing

The importance of examining the skill mix on the ward when planning to change the work methodology was recognized at an early stage in the change process. One study highlighted the need for radical alteration of the skill mix to greatly increase the number of registered nurses, decrease the enrolled nurses and remove all untrained staff. This was needed to ensure staff on the ward had the appropriate skills to implement primary nursing in this particular area (Binnie, 1987).

We were able to manage with less drastic alterations, although, in honesty, we would have found the transition slightly easier if we had perhaps been more ruthless early on. As with any change, one has to consider the local climate when making decisions.

We were influenced by the normative re-educative approach

to instigating change, and the other approaches for managing teams outlined earlier in this chapter. Moving staff who had worked with dedicated enthusiasm on a ward for many years could, we felt, cause disruption as the team rallied round in support against the decision, and it may take years for the perceived perpetrator to be 'forgiven'. Faced with such hostility, the team cohesiveness could break down to the point where moving any of the other factors along the continuum was impossible. We also had concerns about our own abilities to lead a team that had been fragmented by such radical restructuring. All of these factors therefore have to be reviewed to estimate the collective impact.

In order to do this, two final factors need to be explored prior to the introduction of Primary Nursing – leadership style and communications.

FACTOR 7: LEADERSHIP STYLE

The introductory section on change management identified that one of the variables that will influence any change is the change agent, or leader of the change initiative. We recognized the importance of this factor whilst involved in one of our strategies for raising awareness and interest about Primary Nursing, and were visiting a number of other units.

A visit was made to a hospital that seemed to offer the ideal climate for implementing Primary Nursing. It was a new unit with good staffing levels of predominantly trained staff, supportive senior management and an active quality assurance team, and yet the staff seemed apathetic and uninterested, and nothing seemed to be happening. We made comparisons with another unit visited, which, on the surface, had insurmountable difficulties. This was an old Victorian workhouse with poor staffing levels, and yet within this restrictive environment the staff were managing to move towards Primary Nursing. We asked the staff in the second unit what it was that motivated them in the face of such adversity. They all gave the same answer – the Ward Sister. One nurse said 'She's always so cheerful and enthusiastic, and full of good ideas. She works us hard, but it's worth it when you see the results. She really makes us feel we have something worth contributing.'

It made us reflect on the impact that leadership (or lack of it) could have on a team of staff, particularly in relation to developing nursing. General G.S. Patton once commented that leadership is 'The art of getting your subordinates to do the impossible'. Looking around, we began to recognize certain individuals in the profession who seemed to be able to do just this.

A review of the literature, coupled with our own experiences, led us to identify certain approaches and techniques that were useful in helping move along the continuum for this factor in our assessment tool (Peters and Waterman, 1982; Peters and Austin, 1985: Crosby, 1987).

We identified that if Primary Nursing was to be implemented successfully, there was a need to move from an autocratic to a democratic style of leadership. It is only by leading in this way that the staff are enabled to practise within the extended role under the new work methodology.

Approaches useful for providing leadership during the transition to Primary Nursing

First, the leader has a 'vision' of what it is they are trying to achieve. It is this that acts as their primary motivation.

Second, the leader appreciates the role others have to play in helping them turn the vision into reality. Use of the following techniques are instrumental on getting all the staff pulling in the same direction:

- They are eloquent in communicating their vision to all staff.
- They are unswervingly enthusiastic, which infects other staff with the same enthusiasm.
- They recognize the vital role of others in achieving this vision. This means they place genuine value on their colleagues.
- They develop all staff to their full potential. This means they are not threatened by staff who may be more skilled than themselves in certain capacities. (Traditionally, in nursing, this situation led to staff being 'put back in their place' by the hierarchy). Instead, they actively recruit staff who excel in areas in which they themselves are weak.
- They are good listeners, empathic and receptive to new ideas.

- They are consistent and fair.
- They develop team cohesiveness.
- They maintain their professional integrity.

The leadership factor on the assessment tool (Table 4.2) can be one of the most difficult to address, as it is often the individual who is managing the change who is the leader. It is therefore very difficult to be objective about where one falls in relation to leadership style. The most effective way of finding out is to ask the rest of the staff to complete the assessment rating tool independently and anonymously, and see what the rating was for this factor. Another alternative is to explore this issue within a team-building setting, with appropriate facilitation. Another method found to be useful was peer review, with use of some of the personal development rating scales (Bernhard and Walsh, 1981).

This can often be with another colleague of the same grade, but the most effective method (if one is brave enough!) is to ask your subordinates to appraise you in the same way you appraise them. We felt they were the most appropriate individuals to give feedback on criteria such as whether or not staff feel valued, whether the leadership style is autocratic or not. It must be remembered that these approaches were used following interpersonal skills training and team-building ses-sions. Prior to such approaches, we feel such open assessment would have been both threatening and a potential source of conflict.

Some of the 'off the shelf' staff attitude surveys can also act as useful measures of how well the leader is performing, as well as acting as useful benchmarks to track the effect any change in leadership style has on staff.

There is debate in the literature as to whether leaders are born with these skills, or whether they can be taught, although it is widely accepted they can occur at all levels within an organization.

Although sceptical of the concept of previously apathetic and uninterested individuals becoming inspired visionaries within the space of a 4-day management course aimed at developing leadership skills, we found some of these courses offered skill development that greatly enhanced the ability to inspire and develop a team. This was something that was not previously covered on the RGN curriculum, and caused many difficulties in our first Sister's posts, as we were forced to learn these skills through a painful process of trial and error.

We also differentiated between the role of the manager and that of the leader. A helpful definition is explained by Zaleznik (1977):

> Managers relate to people according to the role they play in a sequence of events or in a decision making **process**, while leaders, who are concerned with ideas, relate in more intuitive and empathic ways. The manager's orientation to people, as actors in a sequence of events, deflects his or her attention away from the substance of people's concerns and toward their roles in a process. The distinction is simply between a manager's attention to **how** things get done and a leader's to **what** the events and decisions mean to participants.

It was apparent to us that if we were to demonstrate leadership in creating the climate for changing the work methodology, rather than just managing it, then, in the light of this definition, we would have to incorporate the factor of communication into our assessment tool and implementation plan.

This factor, and strategies used to move it along the continuum on the assessments tool in preparation for the introduction to Primary Nursing, are outlined below.

FACTOR 8: COMMUNICATION

Communication is such an essential factor in moving the other nine factors along their respective continuum on the assessment tool in preparation for the new work methodology that we debated whether or not it should be presented as a separate entity, or integrated into each factor. For ease of presentation, it was decided to incorporate it as a separate Factor on the assessment tool in Table 4.2. This identifies the two ends of the continuum as moving from a minimum position; where the communication networks mainly consisted of passive information passed down the line with no feedback mechanism; to one of active information, with two-way communication.

Organizational communication channels are also included on the assessment tool; with poor channels of organizational communication giving a score at the lower end of the continuum. It is difficult to give staff information if none is passed down to the Ward Sister from higher in the organization, and it difficult to keep others in the organization informed of wa plans and progress if no such mechanisms exist for feeding these into the organization. We noted a feature of this situation to be staff complaining that the only way they found out what was happening in their hospital was via the local press.

The final criterion for assessment within the nine factors was the collective interpersonal skills of the staff. It is important to identify individuals with particular strengths in this area, as well as the weak links in the chain, as the former can be of assistance when attempting to move over to the upper end of the continuum on the assessment tool.

There were therefore three target areas in this factor to address when preparing for the change to Primary Nursing:

- The interpersonal skills of the staff.
- The communication within the ward area.
- The communication channels within the organization.

Approximately 99% of all the problems that presented as restraining forces to our attempts at change arose directly from communication failures at one of these three levels. Strategies used for overcoming this are described below.

Target area 1: interpersonal skills of staff

Many staff were concerned that the expansion of the nursing role, and the greater personal involvement with patients and relatives under the new system, would demand greater coping skills and be more stressful. On exploring reasons why this may be the case, many of us felt unsure that our communication and interpersonal skills were sophisticated enough to deal with the more intimate relationship. As Menzies (1960) identified in her study, nurses are extremely good at 'conversation blocking', which they use as a mechanism against stress. The system of task allocation exacerbates this situation; nurses focusing on a task are less likely to be asked awkward questions. As part of a workshop to raise our awareness of how often we used such techniques, we brainstormed the most popular communication blocking techniques we were all guilty of using. These were:

- I'll come back later.
- I'll be with you in a minute.

- Don't worry about it.
- Ask the Doctor.
- Cheer up!
- I'll make you a nice cup of tea.

Other examples of deficiencies highlighted included, poor body language (particularly talking to the patient from the bottom of the bed), not sitting at the same level as the patient and generally giving the overall impression we hadn't got a second to spare (a condition we referred to as 'busy looking busy').

The other weak area was in the use of closed questions, such as 'Feeling better today, are we?' which limited the patients's response to a straight 'yes' or 'no' when an open question such as 'How are you feeling today?' would encourage the patient to give more information.

We also identified that some of our exchanges with our colleagues left a lot to be desired; most staff were able to cite recent instances when they felt they had been spoken to rudely or aggressively by another member of staff. There was also a feeling that we didn't always pull together as a team as well as we should. This led to us adding team-building to the list of areas we had identified for improvement. However, this area was left until last, as it was felt we needed to improve our communication, assertiveness and counselling skills before embarking on such an initiative. The decision was taken that all staff (including auxiliaries) should be offered an opportunity to be included on these study sessions.

The decision to place such a high emphasis on developing the team was as a result of identifying the benefits of using teams as a method of instigating effective change outlined in the theories we had examined (Kanter, 1983).

Logistics of arranging time out for study leave

Allowing enough staff a full day off the ward to attend study days can be enormously difficult. We have found two ways to achieve this. The first is to set aside 2 weeks a year, outside peak holiday periods, where staff agree that none of them will book annual leave. This potentially gave us ten or more shifts to enable some staff to attend courses and others to cover the ward. We also found that part-time staff valued the study days enough to attend on their days off and take time off in lieu. If there are other wards planning similar events, it may also be possible to arrange to lend a few staff on an exchange basis to cover the study day.

The second method is to involve staff from other areas to make up a viable sized group (it was found that eight to ten staff was an ideal size for such workshops). If using an outside facilitator, charging a fee for staff from other hospitals to attend is one way of covering their expenses, and allowing ward staff to attend for free. We never had any problems selling these places; the workshop topics seemed to reflect a high area of interest for external staff. It is also a good way of networking with other hospitals.

We recommend selecting a venue away from the hospital site if possible, or at least as far away as possible from the ward, to ensure staff attending are not interrupted.

These study days were shown to increase staff confidence and improve their interpersonal skills (Slater, 1987).

Target area 2: communication within the ward area

Improving the staff's interpersonal skills had a positive impact on improving general communications within the ward. The importance of including all other disciplines who are affected by the change to Primary Nursing has already been stressed. Methods that we found helped us to achieve this were:

- *Radically rethinking our approach to managing meetings.* Much time was often wasted and often nothing much seemed to happen as a consequence of the meeting.
- *Circulating notes of all meetings to all 'stakeholders.'* We found that, although some individuals were unable to attend the ward meetings, they appreciated being informed of the content in this way.
- *Including communications as part of the implementation Plan.* This would include a clear action for a named individual, e.g. 'Karen to see Dr Jones re. introduction of Team Nursing by 27.2.92.' All action assignments were always followed up at subsequent meetings for feedback and possible further action.
- *Arranging for a large noticeboard to be set aside specifically for communicating the changes in the work methodology.* The imple-

mentation plan was displayed on this board, along with other relevant information. Use of this board is not recommended until all the verbal communications with staff are completed.

- *Improve the written documentation on the ward.* This is an area that needs addressing prior to the implementation of the new work methodology, as it is extremely difficult to carry out care planned by another member of staff in the absence of any clear written instructions.

Many of our difficulties arose from the fact that the nursing process had been introduced power coercively some years previously, with no proper education for staff. These difficulties were resolved by planning a series of workshops for staff on the nursing process. These were followed by introductory sessions on the more commonly used nursing models. Staff were then given the choice of which model they wished to use.

In the initial months, it was felt that staff had enough change to cope with, and they preferred to opt for one model; 18 months into the project, staff were becoming more creative and examining the use of different models that best fitted the individual patients needs. The final stage was for the team to begin to explore developing their own model. We also recommend setting a standard for the planning of nursing care. This is useful in setting clear requirements and forming the basis of a care plan audit to ensure the criteria are being complied with.

Target area 3: the communication channels within the organization

It is essential to find out what communication systems are already established within the organization and, where appropriate, to use them to communicate the philosophy of Primary Nursing and report on progress. Where team briefing is used, this can prove a useful medium. The hospital newspaper can be a medium for articles about the Primary Nursing and its progress. In the absence of a hospital newspaper, consider starting one. We found this was an effective method for us to establish good links with all areas of the organization at all levels.

Other useful approaches included starting a journals club,

arranging an open lunchtime meeting (free food usually ensured a good attendance!) to explain the new work methodology and allow questions and starting informal support groups with staff from other wards making similar changes to exchange ideas.

In practice, we found it was up to us to develop networks to communicate our aims and objectives, as the organizational channels were extremely poorly developed. However, in one hospital, these were vastly improved with the introduction of total quality management, an approach outlined in Chapter 7.

LEADING THE CHANGE TO PRIMARY NURSING

The assimilation of these nine factors forming the basis of an implementation plan would normally occur in phase 2 – the planning phase – identified under the section on Work Methodology. Drawing on some of the ideas from the literature that we have found useful, the nursing process and on our own experiences, we designed the model below to act as a framework for the process of changing the work methodology on the ward (Figure 5.1.).

The four phases of assessment, planning, implementation and evaluation are shown, with the actions required for each phase. It is shown as a cyclical process, as we have found continuous modification and review of the factors instrumental in changing the work methodology to be necessary. This is because they do not remain static, they are subject to changes as a result of internal and external influences. Even if it is felt that the maximum position is achieved on the assessment tool for a factor, we have found that it can easily slip back towards the lower end of the continuum if it is not continually reviewed using this model.

Each of the nine factors needs to be assessed for their relative position on the assessment tool in Table 4.2. A subjective score is given along the continuum shown. The Team Leader needs to decide where on the continuum each of these factors need to be before introducing Primary Nursing. Ideally, this would mean a score of five for all factors at the upper end of the continuum. Realistically, this may not be possible, but it may be decided that the implementation can still go ahead. For example, it may be that the environmental factor will never be higher than three

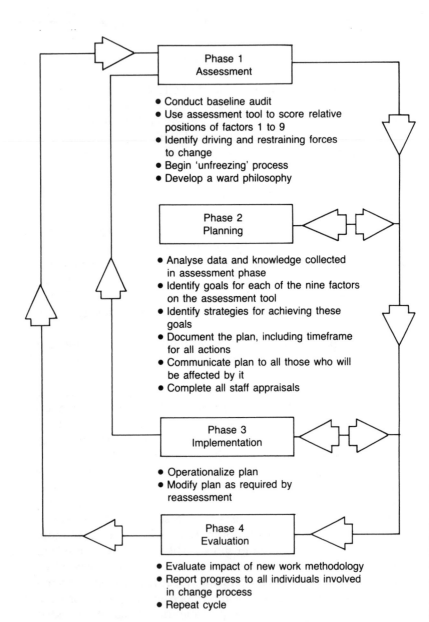

Figure 5.1 An example of an implementation plan for introducing Primary Nursing.

because of local difficulties. However, strategies may be designed to circumnavigate these problems, and it is still feasible to introduce Primary Nursing.

We have stated that we referred to the process of introducing Primary Nursing as changing the work methodology on the ward. This was because of our concern that the term 'Primary Nursing' has been used and abused to describe all manner of initiatives; which, however laudable, do not meet Manthey's original definition (1980). The extent to which nurses in the UK can become truly autonomous and accountable practitioners is limited due to legal restrictions. The notion of 24-hour accountability for a patient, even when the Primary Nurse is off duty, is another element that is difficult to instigate. Given these difficulties, it would be misleading to claim we were 'doing' Primary Nursing within the context of Manthey's definition. However, the changes that were made in the clinical setting as a result of moving towards Primary Nursing, and changing the work methodology, were nevertheless seen by those exposed to the new system as beneficial.

Following the assessment of all nine factors on the tool, and a judgement as to the ideal score for each of these, a plan needs to be formulated with identified goals and strategies for achieving these goals. This involves moving through the stages outlined in the model shown for leading the change towards Primary Nursing in Figure 5.1. This is explained below.

Designing a plan for moving towards Primary Nursing using the nine factors and model

Phase 1: Assessment

This involves moving through each of the activities stated in the above model.

There are two exceptions in the process of repeating the actions in the cycle in the model. These are in the assessment phase and are the baseline audit and the development of a philosophy. After the first cycle, the audit is moved into the evaluation phase as one of the methods to assess the impact of the new work methodology. It is not necessary to develop a new philosophy each time the cycle is repeated, as this is too frequent. We would advise that it is reviewed periodically, as staff may wish to develop and change it. Often, as the factors move over to the right of the assessment tool, attitudes and beliefs can alter as a result of the change.

Phase 2: Planning

This involves working through the actions identified in the model in Figure 5.1 under this phase.

The formulation of an implementation plan, based on the factors in the assessment tool, serves as a useful method of taking some of the more abstract concepts out of the textbooks, and turning them into actionable objectives.

These 'factors' are all interdependent on each other, and, as the systems theory outlines, a change in one factor can influence all the others. For this reason, the factors are not presented as a series of steps of phases, but as a block within the assessment tool to enable an implementation plan to be drawn up to consider all factors simultaneously, assessing the impact certain actions to move one factor to the upper end of the continuum on the assessment tool can have on others.

An example of such an implementation plan is shown in Table 5.1. The theory of change management is not included as a specific area for action, as these will be incorporated into the process of moving all the other factors along the continuum. The headings for actions are necessarily brief, to enable a large amount of information to be presented at once.

We recommend preparing an accompanying project plan, which offers more detail, and the rationale behind the planned approach. In this supplementary written information, each of the factors will have a clear written goal, which must be specific, and measurable. This will include the selection of audit criteria that can be applied at the end of the specified time frame to see if the factor has moved as far as anticipated. For example, in the work methodology factor, the goal may be 'To implement team nursing within 12 months'. Criteria applied at the end of this time could include reviewing the off-duty to see if it is done in teams, and whether or not these are adhered to in practice. In another instance, it may not be practicable to have a fully functioning quality assurance system within the time frame. The goal for the first year may therefore be 'To develop a quality assurance strategy, and improve staff knowledge on the quality assurance tools, Qualpacs, Monitor and Phaneuf'. At the end of the year it will be apparent whether the strategy has been developed, and a brief multiple choice questionnaire on the three tools covered is one way of assessing the effectiveness of the education.

We have found the more detailed project plan useful in helping us communicate to managers, other professionals and new ward staff, the aims and objectives of the change programme. They also proved useful retrospectively as a diary of what had been accomplished.

In referring to the implementation plan (Appendix 5.1), it can be seen that each of the actions has the initials of the individual with responsibility for implementing the action shown. Along the top is a time frame, with the agreed completion dates for the actions are indicated beneath the week number in each month. Where the whole team is to be included, this is indicated by 'All', on the plan. When a group of staff are to attend a study day, 'see rota' indicates that the selected staff are down on the rota for study leave.

All the actions and target dates will be the result of negotiation and agreement between the team and individuals concerned.

Phase 3: Implementation

This involves implementing the plan. Throughout this phase it may be necessary to modify the original plan as a result of ongoing assessment of its effectiveness.

Phase 4: Evaluation

This involves working through the activities listed in the model in Figure 5.1.

At the end of the time frame covered by the implementation plan, the cycle in the implementation model is repeated to generate a new set of goals and actions for the next year. For ease of presentation, the example shown illustrates the actions planned within 12 months. In practice, this plan took approximately 18 months to complete.

This approach (utilizing the model, the implementation plan with project report, based around the nine factors) was developed after some early setbacks in trying to implement Primary Nursing. The mistakes we made were plentiful, but the key pitfalls were as follows.

Pitfalls identified in attempting to move to Primary Nursing without a systematic approach

The first problem was that we found we were so caught up in d. -to-day crisis management that we never seemed to make any long-term plans on how we intended to achieve the change in the work methodology. We always intended to get round to things 'when things were quiet', but we never did, because they never were. By forcing ourselves to stick to a plan with clearly stated goals, make time and stick to deadlines by referring to the implementation plan, we overcame this problem. This is not to say there were not occasions when planning meetings were cancelled because of a cardiac arrest but, on the whole, we found that if we picked a time, and everyone who needed to attend made sure they planned the patient care accordingly, the meeting or educational session usually went ahead. We also found that, by managing our meetings much more effectively, we were able to achieve far more in a shorter space of time.

The second problem was that, initially, we were still functioning under the old culture of 'Sister' being in charge; and tried to do everything alone. This meant that, as well as being exhausting, things were rushed and consequently not as effective as they could have been. It also took a long time to achieve a few objectives. Having a planned, systematic approach helped overcome this problem. This was achieved by negotiating with team members specific responsibilities to share the workload, educational sessions and resource packs, which enabled actions to be carried out more thoroughly, on time and within a much shorter time frame. Input from other disciplines helped even further and had the added advantage of integrating many of the strategies for managing change, such as ownership, raising esteem, increasing motivation and improving communication.

The third problem arose from the second – some of the changes lasted a short while, but seemed to quickly slip back into an old routine as soon as we moved onto something else. With a systematic approach, and all staff championing specific developments, they tended to ensure the momentum continued once the change had been made. Introducing audit criteria into the plan also helped to ensure the change had been 're-frozen' into the new method of working.

The fourth, and by far the biggest problem, was in our inexperience at planning such a major change initiative. Our lack of understanding of the process of change inhibited us further; it was difficult to know where to start, how to sustain the momentum and, finally, whether what we had done had been of benefit. Developing this approach enabled us to manage the transition because of its ability to co-ordinate the whole process. It offered us a framework within which we had the opportunity to consider the impact a particular course of action would have on a myriad of other variables.

This ability to assess and plan all the different factors instrumental in changing to the new work methodology, with consideration for the impact altering one might have on the other, was essential.

For example, 'leadership' is reliant on good communication, both on an interpersonal and organizational level; it is aided by a quality assurance strategy to provide feedback on the impact of their leadership and by the utilization of change management theories to implement the goals of the leader.

Similarly, an effective quality assurance strategy is reliant on effective leaders to establish and maintain it; on the effective interpersonal skills of those within the organization, on a good communication network to collect and disseminate relevant findings and on effective change management to ensure that quality assurance is a dynamic process and that problems identified are effectively resolved.

SUMMARY

These concepts are best summarized in Illustration 5.2.

The work methodology, be it Task Allocation, Team Nursing or Primary Nursing, is shown as the roof of the temple. This is supported by the factors in the pillars below. All too often, staff are disillusioned in their early attempts at changing the work methodology and label the specific approach as a failure. Hence we often hear 'We tried Primary Nursing, but it didn't work'. Using this illustration as an analogy, this is a bit like blaming the roofers for the temple ceiling falling down, when the

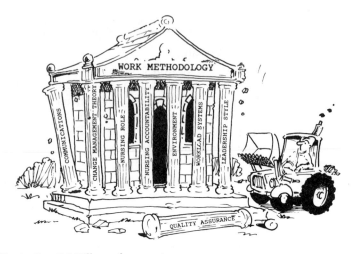

Illustration 5.2 Pillars of support.

builders laid the foundations for the pillars that support the roof on sand.

Understanding the principles of change management was a vital part of implementing the new work methodology, and integral to our quest for quality improvement in clinical practice. However, in spite of our progress, there was still an underlying feeling that 'something' was still missing. We became increasingly frustrated at the inability of 'The System' to provide us with many of the essential components for delivering quality care. In spite of our philosophical meanderings; it still proved virtually impossible to obtain laundry at weekends, an ambulance at a time convenient for a patient or a car parking space in the hospital. Trying to arrange treatments for patients that involved visits to other departments proved a major logistical trauma in terms of arranging appointments, transfer and preparation. It began to dawn on us that, in order to make further quality improvements, we needed to broaden our horizons beyond that of the traditional nursing domain. It was this recognition that led us towards the final piece in the jigsaw in our quest for quality improvement.

Chapters 6 and 7 explore the use of a systematic approach to improving quality that involves the whole organization, commonly referred to as 'total quality management'.

REFERENCES

Bernhard, L.A. and Walsh M. (1981) *Leadership: The Key to the Professionalisation of Nursing*. McGraw Hill, New York, Toronto.

Binnie, A.J. (1987) Primary Nursing, structural changes. *Nursing Times*, **83** (39), 36–7.

Bloore, J. (1984) Manpower planning two, a system from Gloucestershire, *Nursing Times*, **80**, 55–7.

Crosby, P. (1987) *Quality Without Tears*, 3rd edn, McGraw Hill, New York.

Evans, K. and Hind, T. (1987) Getting the message across. *Nursing Times*, **May 6–12**, 40–2

Evans, K. and Slater, J. (1990) Quality assurance, a positive approach. *Nursing Standard*, **February 7th**, 30–2.

Goldstone, L., Ball, J. and Collier, M. (1984) *Criteria for Care*. Newcastle Upon Tyne Polytechnic Products, Newcastle Upon Tyne.

Hertzberg, F. (1968) One more time: how do you motivate employees? *Harvard Business Review*, January – February **46** (1), 53–62.

Kanter, R.B. (1983) *The Change Masters, How People and Companies Succeed through Innovation in the New Corporate era*. Simon and Schuster, New York.

Liddle, B. and Kaye, L. (1991) Quality initiatives, empowering to help. *Nursing Times*, **87** (26), 26–8.

Macdonald, M. (1988) Primary Nursing: is it worth it? *Journal of Advanced Nursing*, **13**, 797–806.

Macintosh, J. (1987) *Nurse Information System*. Paper presented to Doncaster Health Authority, May 1987, Doncaster Health Authority, Doncaster.

Manthey, M. (1980) *The Practice of Primary Nursing*. Blackwell Scientific, Boston.

Menzies, I.E.P. (1960) A case study in the functioning of social systems as a defense against anxiety. *Human Relations*, **13**, 95–121.

Pembrey S. (1989) The development of nursing practice, a new contradiction. *Senior Nurse*, **9** (8), 3–8.

Pembrey, S. (1978) The Role of the Ward Sister in the Management of Nursing. A study of the organisation of nursing on an individualised patient basis. PhD Thesis, University of Edinburgh.

Peters, T. and Austin, N. (1983) *A Passion for Excellence* William Collins Sons & Co. Ltd., Glasgow.

Peters, T.J. and Waterman, R.H. Jr (1982) *In Search of Excellence*, Harper and Row Publishers, New York.

Raven, B.H. and Rubin, J.Z. (1983) *Social Psychology*. John Wiley & Sons Ltd, Chichester.

Rhys-Hearn, C. (1974) Comparison of Rhys-Hearn method of determining nursing staff requirements with the Aberdeen formula. *International Journal of Nursing Studies*, **16** (95), 103.

Savage. B., Widdowson, T. and Wright, T. (1979) Improving the care of the elderly, in *Innovation of Patient Care* (eds D. Towell and C. Harris), Croom and Helm, London.

Slater. J. (1987) *If you are not part of the solution, you are a part of the problem.* Central Nottinghamshire Health Authority, Nottingham.

Slater, J. (1990) Effecting personal effectiveness: assertiveness training for nurses. *Journal of Advanced Nursing*, **15** (3), 337.

Smith, A. (1988) The Yankelonich–McNamara fallacy, in *Super Money.*

Stephens, G.M., Davies, A. and Goldberg, C.B. (1978) *An Evaluation of the Aberdeen formula for Calculating Nurse Establishments in Hospital Wards.* Dyfed Area Health Authority, Carmarthen.

Tappen, R.M. (1989) *Nursing Leadership and Management: Concepts and Practices*, 2nd edn, Davis, Philadelphia.

United Kingdom Central Council for Nursing, Midwifery and Health Visiting (1984). *Code Of Professional Conduct for the Nurse, Midwife and Health Visitor.* UKCC, London.

United Kingdom Central Council for Nursing, Midwifery and Health Visiting (1992). The Scope of Professional Practice. UKCC, London.

Vaughn, B. and Pillmoor, M. (eds) (1989) *Managing Nursing Work.* Scutari Press, London.

Wells, T.J. (1980) *Problems in Geriatric Nursing Care.* Churchill Livingstone, Edinburgh.

Zaleznik, A. (1977) Managers and leaders: are they different? *Harvard Business Review*, May-June, **55** (3), 67–78.

Appendix Table 5.1

Task	April	May	June	July	Aug	Sept	Oct	Nov	Dec	Jan	Feb	March
Goal: Change environment conducive to new philosophy												
• Refurbish old store room for admission interviews (F.H.)		X---	X									
• Order new curtains for beds (S.C.)		X										
• Commence 'open' visiting hours (ALL)			X									
• Install payphone on ward (P.B.)	X											
• Start 'quality circle' for environment (P.M.D., J.C., B.G., E.H., Y.C.)		X										
• Start bursary to fund study leave (L.E.)	X											
• Evaluate goal (P.M.D.)												X
Goal: Implement workload system												
• Review alternative systems (S.T.)	X---	X										
• Discuss with staff and managers (P.M.)			X---	X								
• Draw up implementation strategy (P.M.)				X---	X							
• Implement strategy (P.M., S.T.)							X					
• Evaluate goal (S.T.)								X				
Goal: Improve communications with organization												
• Network and invite staff to ward (ALL)					X---X							
• Start hospital newspaper (S.H., Y.B.)									X			

Month

Appendix Table 5.1 continued

Activity	April (1 2 3 4)	May (1 2 3 4)	June (1 2 3 4)	July (1 2 3 4)	Aug (1 2 3 4)	Sept (1 2 3 4)	Oct (1 2 3 4)	Nov (1 2 3 4)	Dec (1 2 3 4)	Jan (1 2 3 4)	Feb (1 2 3 4)	March (1 2 3 4)
Goal: *Improve communications with team*												
• Communication skills study day (ROTA)	X---X											
• Bereavement counselling study day (ROTA)		X---X										
• Assertiveness training day (ROTA)			X---X									
• Team-building study day (ROTA)												
• Start ward meetings (P.C.)	X X X	X X X X	X X X X	X X X X	X X X X	X X X X	X X X X	X X X X	X X X X	X X X X	X X X X	X X X X
Goal: *Improve communications–written (i.e. care plans)*												
• Care plan audit (G.E.)	X---X	X---X										
• Workshops on nursing process (P.W.)			X---X	X---X								
• Workshops on nursing theory (J.P.)				X---X	X							
• Implement model					X - - - - -	- - - - - -	- - - X					
• Evaluate												
Goal: *Work methodology–Implement team nursing in 1 year*												
• Workshops on primary nursing (P.C.)	X---X	X	X	X								
• Resource packs (T.W.)	X---X											
• Open meeting (K.P.)								X	X	X	X	X
• See multidisciplinary team (A.B./P.T.)					X							
• Develop philosophy (K.P. and ALL)						X---X	X---X					
• Review rota and skill mix (P.C.)										X---X	X---X	
• Select teams (ALL)											X---X	X X X X

Appendix Table 5.1 continued

Schedule chart — Month (each month divided into weeks 1 2 3 4), April through March.

Activity	April	May	June	July	Aug	Sept	Oct	Nov	Dec	Jan	Feb	March
• Information leaflet (R.H.)											X	
• Start primary nursing notice board (M.W.)											X	X
• Team photos and display (J.M.)												X
• Start team nursing (ALL)												
• Evaluate												X
Goal: To prepare staff for new role												
• Workshops/lectures (A.N./P.C.)	X—X											
• Visit other units (see ROTA)			X									
• Primary nursing conference (A.L./I.P.)												
• Local conference (see ROTA)				X								
• Work attachments (see ROTA)				X		X						
• Prepare ward auxilliary role (I.J.)						X						
• Start ward auxilliary role (I.J.)							X					
• Start co-ordinate role (ALL)							X					
• Management course (K.P./P.C.)								X				
• Evaluate								X	X			
Goal: Prepare for increased accountability and autonomy												
• Lecture on code of conduct (region)					X							
• Open meeting (P.C./ALL)						X						
• Resource pack (B.S.)							X					
• Review extended role (M.V.)									X			
• Extended role courses (see ROTA)							X	X				
• Evaluate (K.P.)												X

Month

	April				May				June				July				Aug				Sept				Oct				Nov				Dec				Jan				Feb				March			
	1	2	3	4	1	2	3	4	1	2	3	4	1	2	3	4	1	2	3	4	1	2	3	4	1	2	3	4	1	2	3	4	1	2	3	4	1	2	3	4	1	2	3	4	1	2	3	4
Goal: To devise a QA strategy																																																	
• Literature search (G.E.)	X	–	–	–	–	–	–	–	–	–	–	–	X																																			
• Conference (P.C., P.M.D., G.E.)														X																																		
• Workshops for staff (P.M.D.)																					X	–	–	–	–	–	–	–	X																				
• Devise strategy (G.E.)																													X	–	–	–	X															
• Evaluate (P.M.D.)																																					X											
Goal: To move towards a democratic style of leadership																																																
• Staff attitude survey (L.M.)	X																																															
• Leader to set objectives (P.D.)					X	–	–	–	–	–	–	X																																				
• Staff appraisals (P.D./R.P.)																																																
• Delegate responsibility within new roles (K.P.)													X																																			
• Evaluate																																										X						

6

An introduction to Total Quality Management

A review of the literature in the application of total quality management (TQM) in the management of health care in the UK shows virtually nothing published before 1988. TQM is a new phenomenon within this arena, and one that, in the last few years, has been attracting an increasing amount of interest from managers and professionals within the National Health Service (NHS), as well as the private sector. Finding a clear-cut definition of TQM from the recent publications pertaining to the health service, and from the more prolific texts in applying this approach in industry (where it has been established for significantly longer) proves difficult, as many authors use differing terminology to explain what TQM actually is.

Although the terminology used by authors varies, there are similarities which run through all the various approaches. These are as follows:

Total

TQM involves everyone and everything that happens within the organization, from the part-time cleaners to the Chief Executive, from the specifications for a multi-million-pound hospital to the process of emptying the rubbish bins. There is an understanding that, without this total involvement, the other components of this approach will fail, or have only limited success.

This totality of approach expands across professional and departmental boundaries, as it is widely accepted that a high proportion of quality problems occur at these interfaces. For example, the ward may have an effective system to ensure patients are prepared for theatre, and the theatre an effective system for dealing with the patient on arrival. Yet the system often breaks down when portering staff are unable to transfer patients from the ward to theatre on time. Closer inspection of the problem often reveals a lack of communication between these three areas, and a lack of understanding about the whole process. Each area concentrates on a discrete part, without central co-ordination.

'Total' also refers to the time frame required in adopting this approach, i.e. it is a continuous process or journey, not a short term project or programme.

Quality

The second theme running through the texts on TQM is that of 'Quality', and specifically what this term means, and how it can be consistently achieved. Definitions include:

- Fitness for purpose or use (Juran and Gryna, 1980).
- The totality of features and characteristics of a product or service that bear on its ability to satisfy stated or implied needs (B.S. 4778, 1987).
- The total composite product and service characteristics of marketing, engineering, manufacture and maintenance through which the product and service in use will meet the expectation by the customer (Feigenbaum, 1983).
- Conformance to requirements (Crosby, 1979).

Inherent in all of these definitions (made explicit when placing them in context of the whole approach outlined by these authors) is the connection between the customer and supplier in the quality chain. Hence for all products or services there will be a supplier/customer relationship. Part of this chain will therefore involve determining what it is the customers want, and the suppliers meeting these needs.

'Customer' is a term used in its broadest sense. It also incorporates the next person in line to receive the product or service, as well as the ultimate customer. For example, the porter collecting a patient for theatre from the ward is a 'customer' of this process. He has certain needs, such as the patient being ready for transfer, the appropriate paperwork being complete and being informed in sufficient time to collect the patient. He then becomes a 'supplier' to the theatre, who require him to deliver the patient safely, with appropriate paperwork and at the right time.

Defining 'quality' is an important part of the TQM approach, as it is a word that means different things to different people. This can make the management of quality in large organizations difficult, as for some it means 'excellence' or some kind of unobtainable standard of perfection, whereas others may work from a set of minimum standards, or within an acceptable level of error. For example, a 'quality standard' that 70% of out-patients are seen within 30 minutes may be set. Some may view meeting this goal as a quality service, others may focus on the service the other 30% receive as inadequate.

The definition of quality, and the recognition of the customer/supplier relationship are important to the TQM approach, as it is from these concepts that the third common theme is derived.

Understanding the needs of the customer, recognizing the customer/supplier relationship begins to offer the potential to have some sort of control over the quality of products or services being produced. This is expanded by many experienced in the TQM field, who believe that if enough is understood about the work process it is possible to control, reduce and (some believe) eliminate completely the number of errors that occur within that process.

This leads to another common observation about quality; that it does not just happen of its own accord, it has to be managed.

Management

TQM is concerned with achieving a culture change within the organization. Many authors acknowledge the limitations of the management styles of the 1950s, and the resultant impact on the organizational culture. These were based on macho manage-ment – treating employees as an easily replaceable commodity, a poor attitude towards the customer, accepting waste and error as inevitable (but continually cutting costs) discouraging change, buying from suppliers who offered the cheapest option and competing on price. Such an approach could be successful only if:

- Employees remained subservient.
- Demand exceeded supply.
- Customers' expectations increased very slowly.
- The world-wide situation remained static.

In fact, this was not the case. Britain's share of world trade in manufactured goods fell from 13% in 1960 to 7% in 1980. By 1986 it had fallen still further to 5.5% (Mortiboys, 1990). During this time, there was an increase in the number of competitors, an increase in customer and employee expectations and unpredictable financial systems, all occurring against a backdrop of rapid change. This pattern has been mirrored in the health service, culminating with the introduction of self-governing trusts competing for their share of the health care market. These pressures have caused some managers in the health service to investigate claims that TQM offers an effective solution to these problems, with the Department of Health sponsoring a number of pilot sites in the UK.

'Culture' can be difficult to define in this context, but a useful observation we have made is that it can be reflected by what happens in an organization immediately a problem has been identified. In some organizations, staff will not report the problem. This is usually a result of previous experience, where identifying problems led to an immediate hunt for the 'culprit' or perceived initiator of the problem, with some kind of punitive retribution. In others, staff will not bother to identify problems, as previous experience has shown they are met with apathy and lack of action. An organization practising TQM will acknowledge the problem and those involved in the work process will be given the time and resources necessary to effect an acceptable solution.

The culture change is achieved through a structured framework of implementing quality improvement which incorporates a fundamental change in management style. Common themes running through various approaches include:

- Recognizing the need for effective leadership and management to enable employees to contribute to improving the quality of their work ('Management through people').
- Recognizing the role that all employees can play in improving the quality (or lack of it) of the work process they are involved in.

- Developing a strategy to effect the culture change.
- Developing work-based teams to monitor and improve quality.
- Adopting concepts, tools and techniques that facilitate a greater understanding of the work process (such as statistical process control).
- Improving the customer/supplier relationship.
- Reducing (and for some eliminating completely) errors or mistakes.

These themes crop up continually in the writings of some of the widely acknowledged authorities in this field. Hence it is difficult to attribute some to one specific author, as many appear to adapt and develop the ideas of others. Another difficulty in criticizing some of these approaches is that most of these experts have founded their own consultancy firms, with much of the educational material they supply to clients subsequently being subject to strict copyright agreements, and not available to the general public. This means that the books written are only a part of the material available, with the most recent developments being kept in commercial confidence for the use of clients only.

However, of the better-known authorities in the TQM field, a number have defined certain elements that they believe essential in adopting TQM. These are outlined briefly below. All these authors stress the need to place the key elements of their approach within the context of the totality of their work, as criticizing certain components of the approach in isolation precludes an understanding of the vital interactions of the various concepts, tools and techniques.

Chapter 7 comprises a case study, which explores the implementation of one such approach to examine the application of these concepts within a hospital setting (as opposed to the more common industrial case studies outlined by many of the above authors).

INTRODUCTION TO THE NOTABLE AUTHORITIES ON TQM

W. Edwards Deming

W. Edwards Deming is an American statistician who went to Japan in the late 1940s. He is widely acknowledged as the initiator of the use of statistical quality control measures, which were utilized extensively and successfully by Japanese industry. At the time, Deming preached a message founded on statistics, based on his extensive experience of sampling techniques gained whilst working for the American bureau of the Census.

Drawing on the work of Shewhart (1931), Deming advocated the need to focus on problems of variability in the manufacturing process, and the need to identify their causes. He divides these into 'special causes', which are those effects assignable to individual equipment, machinery or operators, and 'common causes', such as faulty raw materials, which are shared by several operations and are therefore the responsibility of management. He criticizes the approach used in many companies of attempting to look for the cause of chance variation, which typically occurs in the absence of statistical methods. He recommends the use of statistical methods to measure performance in all areas, not just conformance to product specifications. He believes it is not enough to meet specifications, it is necessary to continuously reduce the amount of variation as well. His underlying philosophy is that productivity improves as variability decreases and, as all things vary, statistical methods of quality control are needed.

Deming promotes the need to ensure worker participation in decision making. He blames management for poor quality, stating that they are responsible for 94% of quality problems, and points out that it is management's task to help people work 'smarter, not harder'. A 1986 quote of his, which is perhaps particularly pertinent to the health service, is:

> Failure of management to plan for the future and foresee problems have brought about waste of manpower, of materials and machine time, all of which raise the manufacturers cost and price that the purchaser must pay. The consumer is not always willing to subsidize this waste.

Deming is a severe critic of motivational programmes because he believes that 'doing one's best' is insufficient – one needs to know what to do and have the correct resources to do it. Consumer research is also cited as important, as the needs and requirements of the customer are always changing.

Like many other writers in this field Deming is sceptical of the application of inspection as a method of quality control when used in isolation, as he believes this neither improves quality nor guarantees it. He is also critical of 'acceptable quality levels' (e.g. meeting the required standard 80% of the time). He also notes that simply checking the specifications of incoming materials in insufficient if the material encounters problems in production; it is important that the supplier understands what the material is to be used for.

There were some initial difficulties with Deming's approach, particularly in relation to employee resistance and management uncertainty as to their role in quality improvement, and one criticism was that too much emphasis was placed on the statistical aspects. These problems were addressed by those later Americans who followed Deming to Japan – Juran and Feigenbaum. Deming's later work (1982) also expands beyond statistical methods, including a systematic approach to problem solving – the Deming 'plan, do, check, action' (PDCA) cycle (Figure 6.1). Deming also emphasized the need for senior managers to become actively involved in the organizations' quality improvement programmes.

Deming is well known for his 14 key points, which he cites as essential for the transformation of American industry. These points can apply to any size of organization, as well as to divisions within it, and are:

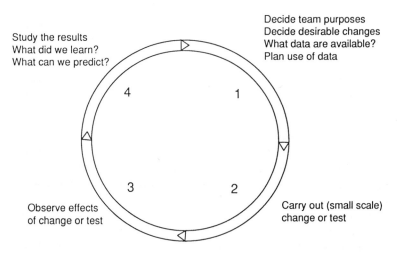

Study the results
What did we learn?
What can we predict?

Decide team purposes
Decide desirable changes
What data are available?
Plan use of data

4

1

3

2

Observe effects
of change or test

Carry out (small scale)
change or test

Figure 6.1 The Deming action cycle.

1. Create constancy of purpose to improve product or service.
2. Adopt the new philosophy.
3. Cease dependence on inspection to achieve quality.
4. End the practice of awarding business on the basis of price tag alone. Instead minimize total cost by working with a single supplier.
5. Improve constantly and for ever every process for planning, production and service.
6. Institute training on the job.
7. Adopt and institute leadership.
8. Drive out fear.
9. Break down barriers between staff areas.
10. Eliminate slogans, exhortations and targets for the workforce.
11. Eliminate numerical quotas for the work force and numerical goals for management.
12. Remove barriers that rob people of pride of workmanship. Eliminate the annual or merit system.
13. Institute vigorous education and self-improvement for everyone.
14. Put everyone in the company to work to accomplish the transformation.

Joseph M. Juran

Juran's background lay in engineering, although other wide-ranging accomplishments include that of university professor. Along with Deming he is credited with influencing the success of Japanese industry in the post-war years. He was invited to Japan in the early 1950s, where he lectured on how to manage for quality. He is noted for dealing with the broad management aspects of quality; identifying the important role of communications, co-ordination of functions and the 'human' element; and stating that an understanding of the human situations associated with the job will go a long way to solving the technical problems and that such an understanding may be prerequisite of a solution.

Juran emphasizes the vital role of management, with the strong message that quality does not happen by accident, it must be planned. In his opinion, 80% of quality problems are caused by management, and he advocates the use of training all managers in quality to enable them to oversee and participate in quality improvement projects. He views the project-by-project approach by problem solving teams as the way to secure overall quality improvement. He stresses the need to include top level management in this process, because he perceives that the major problems in organizations are interdepartmental. He questions the instinctive belief of many top managers that they already know what needs to be done and that training is for others. He also warns of the dangers of departmental goals undermining the company's overall mission. He promotes the use of statistical process control, although warning of this leading to a 'tool-oriented' approach.

His book, *Juran on Planning for Quality* (1988) outlines his structured approach to company-wide planning. He defines a tripartite approach to this: (i) quality planning; (ii) quality control; and (iii) quality improvement. Key elements as part of the implementation of the strategic planning are:

- Identifying customers and their needs.
- Establishing optimal quality goals.
- Creating measurements of quality.
- Planning processes capable of meeting quality goals under operating conditions.
- Producing continuing results in improved market share, premium prices and a reduction in error rates in office and factory.

Juran stresses the importance of securing precision from one's suppliers in achieving a quality product or service and, as such, emphasizes the role of the purchaser. This should include training in methods for rating vendors, with the customer making the investment of time, effort and special skills to help poor vendors improve.

Along with others, he differentiates between the end customer, who receives the final product or service, and other internal and external customers. This incorporates his concept of quality, since 'fitness of use' will need to be ensured at every customer/supplier interface.

He is critical of quality drives based on slogans and exhortations because he does not believe they elicit the required behaviour change. This was usually because such initiatives gave no specific tasks or projects for tackling; did not allocate individual responsibility for doing the necessary tasks; provided no structured process for implementation and did not revise systems used for judging manager performance. He states that 'The recipe for action should consist of 90% substance and 10% exhortation, not the reverse' (Juran, 1988).

Juran lists ten steps to quality improvement:

1. Build awareness of the need and opportunity for development.
2. Set goals for improvement.
3. Organize to reach the goals (establish a quality council, identify problems, select projects, appoint teams, designate facilitators).
4. Provide training.
5. Carry out projects to solve problems.
6. Report progress.
7. Give recognition.
8. Communicate results.
9. Keep score.
10. Maintain momentum by making annual improvement part of the regular systems and processes of the company.

Philip B. Crosby

Philip Crosby is an American with a background in quality control. A quality manager on the first Pershing missile programme, he moved on to ITT, where he eventually became Corporate Vice President and Quality Director. His best selling book, *Quality is Free* was first published in 1979, and he has written a number of other books expanding on his original ideas (Crosby, 1967, 1972, 1984, 1986, 1988, 1990). He has established his own consultancy company, Philip Crosby Associates, which now has 28 offices throughout the world, including the UK.

The Crosby approach to TQM is outlined in Chapter 7, in the case study applying TQM in an NHS setting.

J.S. Oakland

Author of *Total Quality Management* (1989) this British authority on the subject is Professor of TQM at the European Centre for Total Quality Management at the University of Bradford Management Centre. As with many other authors, he stresses the importance of the customer/supplier interface, which he illustrates by the use of a 'quality chain', with the customer and supplier forming the vital links. The chain can therefore be broken at any point if an individual or other essential piece of equipment does not meet requirements. Oakland examines the management of quality through two central concepts: (i) quality of design; and (ii) conformance to design.

Quality of design

This is defined as 'A measure of how well the product or service is designed to meet its purpose'. This involves establishing what the product or service will be used for. The most important feature of the design is the specification. Specifications will also need to be established at each point in the customer/supplier interface.

Quality of conformance to design

This is the extent to which the product or service actually achieves the quality of design. Oakland stresses the need to build statistical process control into the production process, and details this further in his book *Statistical Process Control* (1986). He also emphasizes the need to build prevention into the work process.

Central to achieving the above two factors is the notion of 'work' being a series of interdependent processes, with clear inputs and outputs. Oakland recognizes the need for a co-ordinated, corporate wide framework to integrate these concepts into practice, and utilizes a 13-step implementation plan, as illustrated in Figure 6.2.

Other leading authorities on Quality

There are a number of other notable figures whose thoughts and writing have influenced the development of Total Quality Management in the Industrial Sector. To date, little has been written about the application of these specific approaches in Service Industries perhaps due to the technical nature of some

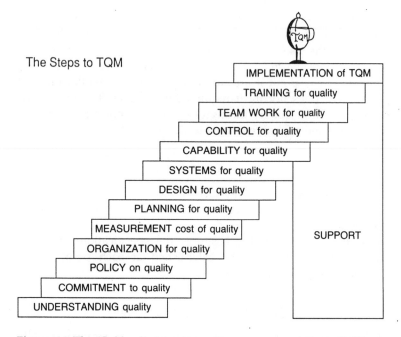

Figure 6.2 The 'Oakland' steps to quality management (from Oakland, 1989).

of the approaches used, which were designed for use specifically in industry. These are briefly mentioned below, including some of the pioneering approaches within the NHS.

Armand V. Feigenbaum

Author of *Total Quality Control* (1983), Feigenbaum defines quality control as:

> An effective system for co-ordinating the quality maintenance and quality improvement efforts of the various groups in an organisation so as to enable production at the most economical levels which allow for full customer satisfaction.

Like other authors in this field, he does not use the term 'quality' as synonymous with 'the best' or 'excellence'. He defines it as 'best for the customer use and selling price'.

His approach expands beyond the mechanics of quality

control to include the human relations aspects of quality management. To this aim, he stresses the need for a channel for communication for product–quality information, and a means of participation for all staff in the overall plant quality programme.

He defines this total quality system as:

> The agreed companywide and plantwide operating work structure, documented in effective, integrated technical and managerial procedures, for guiding the co-ordinated actions of the people, the machines, and the information of the company and plant in the best and most practical ways to assure customer quality satisfaction and economical costs of quality.

The management tool used to achieve this is a 4-step approach that involves:

- Setting quality standards.
- Appraising conformance to these standards.
- Acting when these standards are exceeded.
- Planning for improvements in the standards.

Another key focus of this approach is the notion of 'quality costs', which are divided into:

- Prevention costs (including those of quality planning).
- Appraisal costs (including those of routine inspection).
- Internal failure costs (including those such as re-work or scrap).
- External failure costs (including those generated through warranty and dealing with complaints).

Genichi Taguchi

Taguchi's approach is well known for its 'quadratic loss function', a statistical approach that illustrates that a reduction of variability about the target leads to a decrease in loss and subsequent increase in quality (Taguchi, 1979). In contrast to many other authors, Taguchi (1987) defines the quality of the product as 'The (minimum) loss imparted by the product to society from the time the product is shipped'. This therefore incorporates not only the loss to industry in terms of scrap or rework, maintenance costs, machine downtime and warranty costs, but also the costs to the customer as a result of the products' unreliability, which leads ultimately to further knock-on costs to the manufacturer, as a subsequent fall in market share will inevitably occur.

The focus for this approach is therefore very firmly at the design stage; where rigorous testing minimizes product variability and ensures that quality targets are consistently met. This 'off line' approach to quality control is managed in three stages: (i) system design; (ii) parameter design; and (iii) tolerance design.

This final stage offers a mechanism to further reduce variation within the production process. This is achieved by tightening factors, which are shown to cause variation. It is at this stage the 'loss function' is utilized, with more money being spent on better material or equipment; incorporating the Japanese philosophy of 'invest last' rather than 'invest first'.

Kaoru Ishikawa

Ishikawa is best known for pioneering the quality circle approach in Japan during the 1960s (Ishikawa 1976, 1985). Use of this tool by the Japanese incorporated the education of workers in statistical quality control; an approach slightly different to the use of this tool in the West. The 'seven tools of quality' taught to all employees were:

- Pareto charts.
- Cause and effect diagrams.
- Stratification.
- Check sheets.
- Histograms.
- Scatter diagrams.
- Shewharts control charts and graphs.

Shigo Shingo

Shingo is most famous for his 'poka yoke', 'Defect = 0', or the concept of mistake proofing that appears in many of the other approaches outlined above (Shingo, 1986). The need for statistical sampling is eliminated because whenever a defect occurs the whole production process ceases, the cause is defined and action is taken to correct it. As part of this approach, inspection is used to identify errors before they become defects. This is usually achieved by instrumenting machines with immediate feedback.

Hugh Koch

Hugh Koch is a Management Consultant in Health Care Associate at the Health Service Management Centre at the University of Birmingham. He is one of the few authors who has started to produce work detailing the practicalities of implementing total quality management in a health care setting (Koch and Chapman, 1991; Koch, 1991 a,b).

He has identified a number of difficulties in the application of the concepts to TQM in this setting, namely:

- Lack of top management commitment and vision.
- 'Flavour of the month/year' attitudes.
- Hospital community service culture and management style.
- Poor appreciation of TQM concepts, principles and practices.
- Lack of structure for TQM activities.
- Ineffective leadership.

In Koch's model (Figure 6.3) the following key components are identified. First, the services must be:

- Accessible.
- Effective.
- Acceptable.
- Appropriate (to patients, purchasers and the Department of Health).

Second, the services have to be organized with the appropriate quality input for:

- Clear management commitment, leadership and capabilities.
- Optimum team work and recognition of staff value.
- Implementation of quality techniques (clinical audit, standard-setting, information/monitoring, communications.)
- Monitoring and identification of performance against contract specification and reduction of 'non-conformance'.

This model identifies the need to consider service quality at four levels:

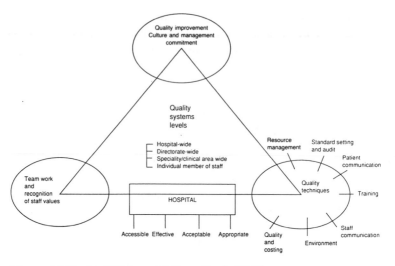

Figure 6.3 Koch's TQM model (from Koch, 1991).

- Hospital-wide.
- Directorate-wide.
- Speciality/clinical-area-wide.
- Individual member of staff.

TQM IN THE HEALTH SERVICE

The texts of the above authors expand on the concepts of their particular approach, and some offer practical advice for imple-, mentation. However, the application of TQM in the health service in the UK is relatively new and (with the notable exception cited above) the majority of texts have not yet diversified to include this area. Other countries, notably Canada and the United States have experimented with TQM in the health care setting (Wilson, 1987; Berwick et al., 1990) but there are difficulties in transferring some of the lessons learnt because of the profound differences between these health care systems and the NHS in the UK.

This cause problems for those wishing to adopt this approach within such an organization. Some may opt to try it for themselves and others to utilize services from the growing number of Management Consultants that offer this facility. Many have recognized the lucrative market offered by the NHS and are keen to get a foothold. There are advantages and disadvantages in using external consultants, some of which are outlined below.

The use of management consultancy firms for the implementation of TQM

It can be useful to have people with expertise helping apply what is an extremely complex and very different approach into a hospital or health care setting, particularly in the early stages. In our experience, these people commonly fall into the following two categories.

First, those with significant experience within the health service, particularly in quality assurance, technology development or financial support, but with limited experience of TQM. Second, those with extensive experience in implementation of TQM in industry, but with limited knowledge of the health service.

There are advantages with the former group, in that they are familiar with the health service and, as such, may be more acceptable to staff, who tend to resist 'non-health professionals'. The difficulty arises when the learning curve of the consultant, with regard to applying TQM in the NHS, is matched by that of their clients. Absence of such experience should be viewed with caution. A good indicator is whether or not the company has in place the structural components associated with their approach to TQM. For example, if they mention company-wide training, have all their employees undertaken this? If they advocate the use of problem-solving teams, how many do they have and what kinds of problems have they solved? If they refer to the 'cost of quality', when did their company last use this tool?

There are advantages in using the second group of consultants if they have a proven track record of implementing TQM in an industrial setting. This gives an assurance that the approach has been validated elsewhere, and can work. The difficulty arises in deciding whether or not the approach is 'culturally acceptable' to the NHS, and whether it is adaptable to this setting. We use the term guardedly, as one of the aims of TQM is to change the organizational culture, and one needs to differentiate between what is a threat to the traditional style of management and what could be a genuine difficulty in transferring a particular tool or concept to a health care environment.

Consultants also offer a variety of educational packages, for all levels of the organization, and their experience in teaching these courses. This can be an advantage when one considers the time, effort and money that would need to go into producing such packages from inception. However, these materials must be suitable for the target groups at the outset.

There are major advantages to developing a successful 'in-house' package in those cases where there is sufficient in-house expertise. It is geared to local needs; it is taught by those who have developed it, giving a strong commitment to making it work; it can prove cost-effective, and hospitals who develop such a package have the option of competing on the consultancy market themselves and generating income.

An obstacle to creating such a package is in avoiding infringement of copyright when utilizing work previously published by specialists in this field. Consultancy companies are fiercely protective of their materials and there are already cases of substantial payments awarded for use of their material without permission in the industrial sector.

A good consultancy firm will aim to promote self-sufficiency for the client developing TQM. This should involve developing local staff to enable them to teach these courses. It can be advantageous in the early stages for the training at executive board level to be done by someone well versed in the principles of TQM from outside the organization. First, it is essential to gain the commitment and good understanding of senior executives if TQM is to be adopted throughout the organization (and few in-house course facilitators would relish the thought of running their first course with the top management in the hospital if they have limited practical experience in this field). Second, the consultant can work with the executive board to create a local framework for managing quality. Third, if the executive board has selected consultants in whom they have confidence and respect, they are likely to be receptive to their suggestions, working in a partnership to adapt the approach to local needs.

From our experience, we would recommend that the consultant and client need to work together in drawing up the specifications for the TQM approach. There is the potential for difficulties to arise if a particular approach is too rigid to incorporate the local culture. Similarly, there is a danger of the client drawing up a list of specifications for a TQM approach from a very scant knowledge of what is required, rather than encouraging input from the expertise of the consultant at the specification stage. The traditional approach of selecting a number of consultants to present a short synopsis to a panel, who then 'choose' one at the end of a day's interviewing is beset with problems. It is crucial that time and effort is dedicated to select the right approach to fit with the hospital culture, not least because of the significant resources this will entail.

A major disadvantage in employing external consultants is the cost. TQM is not a short-term project, it is a long-term process. Similarly, developing a home-grown version can incur significant costs, even though these may be hidden in terms of staff time devoted to the project. Funding therefore needs to be considered on an ongoing basis. Considerable financial benefits can be gained from this approach, but an initial investment of cash is required to start the process of implementation, of which the staff training budget represents a high proportion of the cost.

Once the particular approach (or combination of approaches) to TQM has been determined, the process of implementation begins. In our experience, the difficulties of this challenge were exacerbated by the lack of practical advice available on where to begin, what to do and how to sustain the momentum of such an extensive process.

The textbooks talk about concepts such as 'commitment', 'involvement', 'education', 'error costs' and 'measurement', all of which we could appreciate and comprehend. What we needed to know was how, in an average NHS hospital, these concepts can be realized in practice. For example, how does one gain commitment? how can it be sustained? how can we involve everybody and co-ordinate their involvement in a systematic way? what are the logistics of educating everybody? what are we going to teach them? how much are all the errors in our processes costing us? how do we reduce these costs? how and what should we measure? what do we do with the measurement data? These were just some of the myriad questions that faced us at the time. They are also typical of the questions often posed to us from others considering adopting this approach.

In an attempt to provide an insight into what can be involved in the implementation of TQM in a health service setting, Chapter 7 outlines a case study based on our personal experiences. The purpose of outlining how we did it is to give others considering adopting TQM an appreciation of what this can entail, some of the pitfalls we identified and some general ideas that may be considered useful. As noted in the introduction to this chapter, common themes run through all approaches to TQM. These include addressing the practicalities of developing a structure to manage quality, embarking on organization-wide education, introducing measurement, securing and demonstrating management commitment, solving problems and giving recognition to staff and raising awareness. All approaches will have to face these issues, albeit under a different 'handle'. The Crosby approach to TQM is cited in this case study purely because it was the consultancy company appointed at the time. It is not the intention to recommend this approach over any other; due to lack of knowledge with implementing any other approaches in practice. For this reason, no comparable critiques of other approaches are offered, as the intention is to offer practical suggestions for the implementation of TQM rather than an 'armchair critique' of the different theories.

AN INTRODUCTION TO THE CROSBY APPROACH FOR TQM

The philosophical basis for Crosby's approach is based around five central concepts, namely 'All work is a process' (explained in detail in Chapter 1) and what he referred to as 'the four absolutes' of quality management. Crosby does not use the term TQM but refers to his approach as the quality improvement process (QIP). This is subtly different to the common definitions of TQM and explained on page 233.

The four absolutes are the answers to four questions that Crosby believes it is absolutely essential to answer concerning quality. These are:

- What is the definition of quality?
- How is it achieved?
- What is the performance standard?
- How can it be measured?

The answers to these questions and their application within a health service context, are explored below.

What is the definition of Quality?

A typical list of common responses when posing this question to NHS staff are:

- Excellence.
- Expensive.
- Durability.
- Luxury.
- Reliability.
- Marks and Spencer.

It can be appreciated from this list that there are two major problems when attempting to use such definitions in the NHS. First, people's perceptions of 'quality' vary widely. This can make it difficult when addressing quality issues because differing interpretations of the concept of quality can prove a barrier to communications. Second, such definitions are subjective and unquantifiable, making it difficult to measure quality. It is difficult to assess whether a service is more 'excellent' or more 'luxurious' this year than last year.

To generate further discussion, staff were asked to consider a standard issue hospital chair (the plastic stacking type) and debate whether it was an example of a 'quality' chair. This added a further dimension to the debate. It was agreed that the chair was no antique, but this raised the issue of whether or not a 3-foot wide, leather, £500 chair was a desirable substitute. It was decided not, on the grounds it was not easy to clean, was too expensive and required too much storage space. An important factor in judging the quality of the chair was therefore what it was intended to be used for. A list of requirements was drawn up for a chair that was only intended to be sat on for periods of no more than 2 hours (such as visiting times or meetings) and which could be stored between use due to limited space.

The revised verdict on the chair was that it was a quality product, based on these new criteria. It was relatively easy to list quality requirements for a product such as a chair, but there were concerns this would not be as easy in a service-oriented organization such as the NHS.

Referring back to the original list of definitions, we picked up on the use of 'Marks and Spencer' as being synonymous with quality. Staff brainstormed a list of criteria that they believed were important in judging a service organization (such as shops, banks or restaurants) to be one that offered good quality. These included:

- Pleasant, helpful staff.
- Staff with good knowledge about the service who could give informed advice (for example, if things were delayed, how long the customer would have to wait; specific expertise on the service offered).
- Environment (for example, tasteful decor, furnishing and carpets in good repair, cleanliness).
- Good car parking facilities.
- Prompt service (staff felt they should not have to wait more than 5 minutes in a bank or shop queue).
- A wide choice of goods or services.
- Clear signposting.
- Customer complaints dealt with courteously and efficiently, with easy access to senior management.
- Value for money.
- Open at convenient hours.
- Privacy (many disliked the communal changing rooms in some clothes stores).

Hence it was possible to establish criteria for services as well as products. Using this list of criteria, we scored our own hospitals' performance using a score of 1 to 10, and noted that there was considerable scope for improvement. It was identified that part of the process for establishing criteria would entail determining the expectations of the customer, which could be done via market research.

There were some difficulties when transferring this approach to the NHS. For example, when going out for a meal, the customer has clear expectations of the restaurant and the food, based on a set of known requirements. When coming into hospital, the majority of patients are unaware of what many of their requirements are. Some are easy to establish, for example, being treated courteously, short waiting times, environmental and comfort factors (the 'desired' requirements). However, patients are unable to define other requirements of the service they receive, such as the technical and professional aspects of their care. Most would not be able to identify the requirements of a 'quality' appendicectomy, or judge the 'quality' of the equipment used to treat them. In this instance, the professionals involved in treating the patient need to define these 'needed' requirements for them. This is possible if one refers back to the concept 'all work is a process'. What actually happens to a patient on admission to hospital is a series of many different processes (for example, admission, diagnosis, treatments and discharge). The requirements of each of the processes (both from the perspective of the patient and the professional) can be identified using the process model worksheet. Crosby acknowledges this by differentiating between 'desired', 'needed' and 'mandatory', e.g. (Government and professionally mandated) requirements for each process.

In view of the lack of knowledge the majority of the public have about the processes in hospital, there are difficulties in applying definitions of quality such as 'satisfying the customer' or 'exceeding customer expectations'. We identified that many patients have differing expectations of the service, and they are only able to judge the care in comparison to treatment received in other hospitals. A patient who waits 4 hours in a Casualty in one hospital, and 2 hours in another might therefore consider the second hospital as having a reasonable waiting time, as they expected to wait 4 hours. This presents enormous problems when trying to determine patient satisfaction levels using survey techniques.

Staff also identified that, often, patient satisfaction with their care did not always concur with what staff perceived as 'quality' care. Examples were given of a patient whose surgical treatment was a technical success, and saved his life. He wrote a letter of complaint about the poor quality of service in the hospital because the food was not to his liking, staff kept waking him up at night to take his blood pressure and a pair of his pyjamas had gone missing. At the other end of the scale was a patient whose treatment and resultant problems resembled a report to the health service ombudsman. Yet she thought her care was excellent because 'everyone has been so kind'.

Crosby's first absolute of quality management

The definition of quality is conformance to requirements.

If management wants people to 'do it right the first time', then employees need to know what 'it' is, and have the resources to achieve 'it.' 'It' is the requirements that are essential to the process, as identified through the process model worksheet (see Figure 1.2). The agreement of these requirements between all of those involved in the process is an essential part in maintaining a quality service. Once the requirements are established clearly, the process of auditing them to see if they are being met becomes possible.

What is the system for ensuring Quality?

The system commonly adopted to ensure quality by many industrial companies in the US and the UK in the 1950s was that of 'inspection', which fell under the remit of the quality control department. Quality control involved checking the product as it came off the production line to identify any faulty goods, which were either rejected or 'fixed' by a group of staff especially employed for this purpose. Along with this approach arose the notion of 'acceptable quality levels.' These were laid down by management, or the customer, and stipulated the accepted level of faulty goods. For example, 90% of chocolates produced would meet the specifications.

In recent years, many companies have identified several difficulties associated with this approach:

- *It is retrospective*. This causes difficulties in managing quality, since errors are only identified *after* they have occurred.
- *It is expensive*. Extra expense is incurred in employing staff to check the product; employing others to fix it; and in the wasted materials.
- *It generates a 'fix it' approach to errors*. Fixing mistakes after they occur alleviates the symptoms of poor quality (in that they are not passed on to the customer) but does not tackle the root cause of why the problem arose in the first place.
- *It is threatening for staff*. Typically, the knowledge that the quality control team were coming on a visit to a division would be viewed with trepidation. As one worker observed 'We put as much time and effort into hiding our mistakes as the Quality Manager does in trying to find them.'

The whole cultural climate created by such an approach is one based on fear of management. It also places the responsibility for detecting errors in the hands of those who have limited knowledge of the work process that is producing the errors, rather than with those who have the greatest insight as to why problems may arise, namely the workers involved in the process.

In view of these limitations, it can be appreciated that such an approach could have even greater difficulties when applied to the NHS, where the 'product' is not an inanimate object but a health service that is delivered to patients.

In spite of this, many approaches to quality assurance in the NHS still retained these four weaknesses. In one respect, the rush for audit was putting the cart before the horse. The tools identified weaknesses in the service and where errors were made (such as in monitoring customer complaints) but no effective method for solving these problems had been established prior to such an audit. This undermined the usefulness of many of the quality assurance tools, with some staff dismissing them as a waste of time. In fact, it was not the tools themselves that were at fault. Audit is an essential part of quality management. The reason staff became disillusioned was because of the way in which they were implemented and used by management. There is absolutely no point in spending time and money on audit if nothing improves as a result.

Crosby's second absolute of quality

The system for causing quality is prevention of mistakes.

This changes the focus from detecting mistakes after they have occurred to preventing them from occurring in the first place. Crosby believes this can be achieved by close analysis of the work process (by use of the tools and techniques) and building prevention into the process itself. Such an approach can only be fully realized by empowering staff to improve their work, as they are in the unique position of being able to identify weaknesses and offering solutions.

What is the performance standard?

In one of our workshops, staff were asked to consider the application of 'acceptable quality levels', in relation to three health service work processes: (i) amputating a patient's leg; (ii) ensuring patients received the lunch they ordered; and (iii) filling in forms correctly.

It was unanimously agreed that there was no room for error in the case of the patient having a leg amputated. It was expected that, in 100% of cases, the correct leg would be amputated, with all the necessary requirements for this process being met.

The process of delivering the correct meal to the correct patient created some debate. It was accepted that there were occasions when this did not happen. Some nurses raised the concern that this could be detrimental to the patient, for example, a diabetic patient receiving a non-diabetic meal. In view of this it was generally accepted that, in 100% of cases, the patient should receive the correct meal.

The process of filling in forms was viewed as tedious, which staff rated as a low priority. Many felt that there were too many forms, and filling them in detracted from time spent in direct patient care. Staff were then asked how often they were on the receiving end of incomplete paperwork, which brought forth a flood of complaints. For example, the pathology and X-ray departments estimated that between 20% and 30% of the request forms they received were incomplete or inaccurate. On exploring the problem further, nursing and medical staff were largely ignorant of the 'hassle' (a word that was used frequently) they caused these areas when sending poorly completed forms. A common complaint was that parts of the form were perceived as irrelevant to the person filling them in. This illustrated the clear lack of agreed requirements on the form design. As staff began to appreciate the significance of various forms, the 'acceptable quality level' began to change. It was agreed that filling in the forms properly was not technically difficult, and there was no real excuse for not achieving 100% compliance.

In terms of the performance standard for staff when doing their work, and the impact not meeting these standards could have on the patient, it was agreed that staff should 'get it right the first time'. An advantage to meeting this standard was identified in the reduction of 'hassle' and time wasted doing things over again. As we noted, we were always too busy to fill out forms properly, but we always had to find time to do them again when returned to us.

Crosbys' third absolute of quality management

The performance standard is zero defects.

Prior to completing the educational courses, staff found the wording rather Americanized. In spite of this, they grasped the concept when explored further, although 'Do it right first time' was felt to be a more acceptable alternative.

'Zero defects' is the most commonly misunderstood of Crosby's concepts. Deming categorizes it along with motivational programmes, and others misunderstand it to mean 'perfection', and therefore view it as unachievable.

The educational material is clear that this is not the case. The purpose of zero defects is to create an attitude within the staff that no amount of non-conformance is acceptable. (Crosby uses the term 'non-conformance' when his first absolute of 'conformance to requirements' is not met, i.e. there is a mistake or an error. These are the requirements as defined in the process model worksheet by the customers and suppliers of the process. They will therefore be both achievable and measurable.)

For example, staff have a 'zero defects' standard on the prescribing and administration of drugs, in that it is appreciated that no amount of error is acceptable. This does not mean that drug errors never occur. However, there is an attitude that, if they do occur, appropriate steps are taken to decrease the likelihood of the same mistake being made again. This philosophy is expanded to all work processes (including filling in forms!). Many of us identified that we had the attitude that many of the things that caused us hassle were inevitable and insoluble. We constantly received 'non-conforming' equipment or services from other departments and fixed it ourselves, rather than discussing the problem with the department concerned. This seemed to be a cultural problem within our organization, as we tolerated things at work that would not be tolerated in our private lives. However, such an attitude is self-perpetuating, as the problems that caused us hassle were never solved. We needed to work at making sure things were done correctly the first time.

How can Quality be measured?

There were other consequences of not identifying and meeting requirements, not building prevention into our work processes and not 'getting it right' the first time. Apart from the hassle, there was also a cost in terms of time and money. Staff were asked how much of their time was spent sorting out problems that arose because things had not been done right the first time, or 'fire fighting'; estimates ranged from 10 to 90%. Ward Sisters and middle managers typically stated the highest figures. We built up a picture of what we called 'the Monday morning syndrome'.

The Monday morning syndrome

It is Monday lunchtime. The Doctors are stressed because the ward round was delayed for 20 minutes waiting for some X-rays to be found; theatre is running late, which means cancelling cases; there are no empty beds and they spent an hour ringing round to try and find one for an acute admission.

The Charge Nurse is stressed because there were not enough breakfasts for the new admissions and it took 20 minutes to get some sent up from the kitchen; stock items on the drug trolley had run out and it took an hour to complete the drug round as a result; there was no clean laundry and a nurse had to go borrowing from other wards.

The staff nurse is stressed because two admissions arrived that no one had told her were expected; and an ambulance arrived to transfer a patient, but a chair had been booked instead of a stretcher. As a result it took 45 minutes to re-book another ambulance.

The enrolled nurse is annoyed because she had an appointment with the unit manager at 10 a.m. and waited 30 minutes outside her office before being told she was too busy to see her today.

The auxiliary is tired because she has made three trips to the kitchen, two trips to pharmacy, searched the ward and department for missing X-rays and been round all the wards borrowing linen.

Staff caught up in such a scenario are not doing the job they are employed to do for a significant proportion of their time. Staffing is the largest single expenditure within the hospital budget and yet, as a result of things not happening in the way they are supposed to, this resource is not used to its full potential.

Financially, this can prove expensive. One hospital calculated that, due to the pharmacy not being able to meet its requirements, nurses regularly had to 'nip down' to pharmacy to collect urgent drugs or drugs for patients who were awaiting discharge. These 'nips' equated to two whole time equivalent nurses when they were multiplied up for an average week (mean times taken to walk backwards and forwards to pharmacy in a large hospital multiplied by the total number of nurses 'nipping').

Many managers cited examples of meetings starting late. If one considers the case of ten managers waiting 12 minutes for a meeting to start, this represents 2 hours of management time that is wasted per meeting. Multiplied by the number of late meetings over a year, it can be appreciated there is a significant cost to the organization.

There are other financial costs in the Monday morning scenario. Cancelled theatre lists evoke costs because, in the majority of cases, the patients are occupying a hospital bed in anticipation of their operation, and many will have had X-rays, blood tests and other pre-operative routine procedures. This is on top of the daily cost of keeping a patient in an NHS bed. All this money is wasted in the event of a cancellation. Then there is the added cost of re-admitting the patient at a later date. Mistakes made on ambulance bookings, particularly in the event of an ambulance having to leave without a patient, are also wasteful.

Crosby's fourth absolute of quality management

The measurement of quality is the price of non-conformance

Crosby stresses that for every error there is a cost, either in re-work, waste (either of time, materials or both) and often a knock-on effect in other areas. He estimates that such error costs can be as high as 40% of the annual budget in service industries. Preliminary surveys in the NHS show this to be between 23 and 30% of the annual budget. The purpose of calculating a price for these errors is two-fold.

First, it is an effective method for gaining management attention for a problem. In terms of impact, nurses constantly voicing concerns about the contents of CSSD packs generates less response than a report showing the amount of CSSD waste, with supporting data, calculated as costing £25,000 per annum.

Second, it acts as a baseline measure to determine how the quality improvement process is working. It is also important to build on measurement techniques currently being utilized within the hospital, such as medical audit and the various quality assurance tools. The cost of quality should be viewed as an adjunct to such tools, not as a replacement. In practice, we also found the tools and techniques outlined in Chapter 1 helpful in developing clinical audit.

PRELIMINARY SUMMARY

Crosby's four absolutes of quality management are:

- The definition of quality = conformance to requirements.
- The system for quality = prevention.
- The performance standard = zero defects.
- The measurement of quality = the price of non-conformance.

Underpinning these is the concept that 'All work is a process, a series of actions that produces a result.'

The integration of these concepts into the culture of an organization is managed through an implementation framework, as shown in Figure 6.4. Here, the concepts are supported by commitment, teamwork and systems, which are divided into 14 steps. These are, in turn, supported by the tools and techniques, some of which are outlined in Chapter 1.

Crosby views his 14 steps as essential to establishing a successful quality improvement process, in conjunction with his other concepts. In practice, we found the term 'steps' misleading, as it implied that they be done in sequence and, although the educational material stressed this was not the case, it confused some staff. Eight of the steps are addressed initially, and (as demonstrated through the theories of change in Chapter 5), they need to be considered in relation to their influence on other steps. These steps, and the practical aspects of implementation, will therefore be discussed in the order in which we tackled them, rather than chronological order. For each step we define the purpose, discuss how it was approached and implemented, and identify specific examples of what worked well and what presented problems.

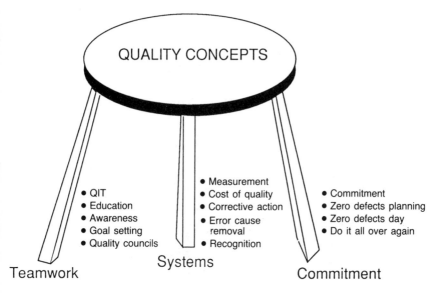

Figure 6.4 The 'Crosby' approach to quality management. QIT = quality improvement team.

In order to implement the steps, a structure for managing quality within the organization needs to be established. General guide-lines for doing this, based on our experiences, are outlined below.

ESTABLISHING A STRUCTURE FOR QUALITY IMPROVEMENT

In spite of the success of some of our earlier attempts at initiatives with quality as a central theme, such as quality assurance, quality circles, setting standards and 'Personalizing the service', there were several common problems that we identified with these approaches. Our frustrations at such problems are summarized in Illustration 6.1, and were:

- Many of them started well, but seemed to run out of steam after a while.
- Many of the staff involved in these projects had a great deal of enthusiasm and commitment but were disadvantaged by having little personal power within the organization. The role of the manager was therefore crucial in realizing the aims of

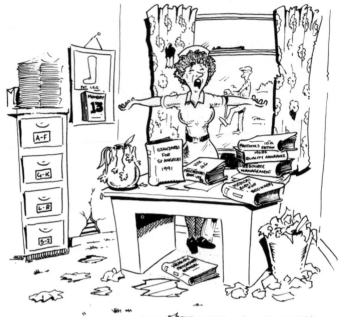

"IVE BEEN RESOURCE MANAGED, QUALITY ASSURED, NURSING STANDARDED, MEDICALLY AUDITED, AND YET I STILL CAN'T GET THE BINS EMPTIED, OR A PILLOW CASE ON A BANK HOLIDAY MONDAY."

Illustration 6.1 Quality assured?

their particular initiative. There were examples of this not being given, with resultant disillusionment and loss of morale.

- Medical staff seldom got involved in these initiatives.
- Funding to support such initiatives was limited.
- There was little central co-ordination, hence different areas often worked on similar problems and work was duplicated rather than shared.
- Quality circles, standard-setting, medical and nursing audit tended to reinforce departmental and professional boundaries because they were predominantly interprofessional or inter-departmental. In practice, realization of these initiatives was dependent on factors outside the control of these groups. For example, nurses could spend months developing a superb discharge standard, but if the medical staff give only 5

minutes notice of a patient's discharge, this standard can never be met. Similarly, medical audit may determine discharge summaries should reach the patient's General Practitioner within 7 days of discharge, but this cannot be met without co-operation from the medical secretaries.

• There was no forum where staff could raise problems identified through such initiatives, or for senior management to learn what these were to enable them to take action.

These problems arose from the traditional approach (or lack of one), to the process of managing quality in hospitals; it was just accepted that 'quality' would happen. Hence no clear direction was given from senior management, there was no budget allocated for it and there was no one individual with a responsibility to co-ordinate these initiatives.

This changed slowly due to a combination of initiatives. Political pressure was pushing quality as an important issue against a backlash of criticism of cost-cutting and growing waiting lists, culminating in the white paper *Working for Patients*. Hospitals were encouraged to prepare 'quality strategies' and a number of individuals suddenly found themselves with 'quality manager' added to their title. Many of these were disadvantaged by the fact the new role was not integrated into the hierarchical structure of the hospital, and had therefore to rely purely on personal power as the post had no position or financial power. They were therefore totally reliant on the support of senior management and consultant medical staff in implementing any quality initiative. With such posts being new within the health service, many post-holders were unsure exactly what was expected of these roles.

Crosby recognized the difficulty of such a structure for managing quality. Like all the other authors in this field, he stresses that management commitment to making quality happen is absolutely essential. Quality should be led, by example, from the top of the organization. This includes having the quality manager on the Executive Board. As he points out, quality is as serious an issue as finance, therefore both need representation on the board.

There were some general guide-lines we found useful when developing an organizational structure for managing quality. These were as follows:

Identify the structure

The structure for managing quality should align as closely as possible to the current hierarchical structure.

This is important, as it is essential that line managers take responsibility for quality in their area. At first we expressed concerns about this, as there were individuals who we knew would be unhappy with this arrangement. However, the alternative (which is to give interested individuals lower down the organization responsibility for quality) is fraught with difficulties. Essentially, the end result is a series of poorly co-ordinated initiatives, of the kind outlined above. In our experience, the most resistant line managers have more difficulty subverting the efforts of quality improvement if they are given an active part in its implementation and it is included as part of their objectives. Furthermore, staff look to management involvement for an example that things are changing. A common criticism by staff of many of the initiative-led approaches to quality was that if it was really that important, why weren't there any managers or senior medical staff actively involved?

Convene a steering committee

The steering committee guides the quality improvement process.

Ideally, this should be driven from the top of the organization as a demonstration of management commitment, and chaired by the Chief Executive. Another alternative is that a subgroup of Executive Board members joins with other individuals from within the organization, who have significant influence within it, and those with any specialist knowledge in quality to make up the steering group.

It is vital that the steering committee has sufficient authority to allocate funds and make decisions. Initially, due to the volume of work involved, senior management may be tempted to create a steering committee of middle managers who report directly to them. This creates problems, as staff view it as a lack of commitment, resulting in the quality improvement process being perceived as a low priority. Second, if the steering committee has to refer continually to another group to authorize its decisions, things take longer to implement and the group may be regarded by many as a 'toothless watch-dog'.

Devise an implementation structure

The steering committee devises the structure for implementing the quality improvement process throughout the rest of the organization.

The structure recommended is shown in Figure 6.5, which is a modification of the model used in practice. This was altered due to some of the difficulties of the original structure. Here it can be seen that a number of quality improvement teams (QITs) are the functional unit for implementing the quality improvement process within a given area. The steering committee needs to decide how best to divide up the organization, defining the areas to be represented by each QIT. In our experience, a manageable unit for a quality improvement team is roughly 400 whole time equivalent staff.

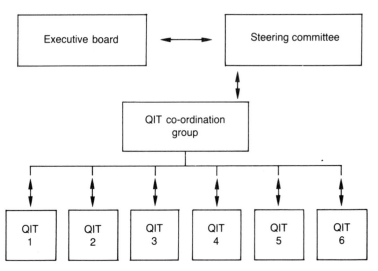

Figure 6.5 A structural framework for the quality improvement process.

Dividing the organization into Quality Improvement Teams

There are several ways to divide the organization:

- *It can be split through professional groups.* For example, a QIT consisting of medical staff is responsible for all the medical staff in the hospital. We would not recommend this approach because it reinforces the professional boundaries that the quality improvement process is trying to overcome.
- *It can be split through geographical location.* Such an approach can be advantageous in a large organization, particularly if divided into different blocks or working across several sites.
- *It can be split through clinical specialties.* For example, the medical unit, surgical unit, X-ray unit, etc. all have their own QIT. This can help break down professional boundaries because the QIT will be multidisciplinary. However, care needs to be taken not to enhance departmental boundaries, such as, for example, creating barriers between the surgical unit and theatres. One way of overcoming this is to have cross-speciality QITs that are heavily dependent on each other in solving work-related problems, as in the case of surgery and theatres or medicine and coronary care.

Once the split has been made (advisedly with consultation with the heads of department and senior members of the professional staff) the senior managers identify members of the QIT. The role of the steering group is then to provide guidance and support for the QITs.

Co-ordinating the Quality Improvement Teams

Within a larger organization, we found there was a need to co-ordinate the efforts of the quality improvement teams and provide a forum where they can share experiences, report on progress and identify problems that require resolution at steering committee level. This should be co-ordinated by the Quality Manager. Monthly meetings of the Chairs of all the QITs are recommended as an effective approach (this group is therefore also identified in Figure 6.5).

Initially, we baulked at what appeared to be another bureaucratic structure, and the amount of work involved in creating it. In practice, it is virtually impossible to manage a cultural change of the magnitude of TQM without some sort of structural framework. Without it, there is no central direction or control, no access to the system for all members of staff and there is a danger that staff work on projects that are at odds with the overall management goals for the organization. Without it, there is no total quality management.

REFERENCES

Berwick, D.M., Glanton, G.A. and Roessner, J. (1990) *Curing Health Care: New strategies for quality improvement*, Jossey Bass Inc., San Francisco.

BS 4778 (1987) *Quality Vocabulary: Part 1 – International Terms (ISO 8402 (1986)*, HMSO, London.

Crosby, P.B. (1967) *Cutting the Cost of Quality*, USA Quality College Bookstore, Orlando, Florida.

Crosby, P.B. (1972) *The Art of Getting Your Own Sweet Way*, McGraw-Hill Book Co., New York.

Crosby, P.B. (1979) *Quality is Free*, McGraw-Hill Book Co., New York.

Crosby, P.B. (1984) *Quality Without Tears*, McGraw-Hill Book Co., New York.

Crosby, P.B. (1986) *Running Things: The art of making things happen*, McGraw-Hill Book Co., New York.

Crosby, P.B. (1988) *The Eternally Successful Organization: The Art of Corporate Wellness*, McGraw-Hill Book Co., New York.

Crosby, P.B. (1990) *Leading: The Art of Becoming an Executive*, McGraw-Hill Book Co., New York.

Deming, W.E. (1982) *Quality, Productivity and Competitive Position*, MIT Center for Advanced Engineering Study, Cambridge, Massachusetts.

Deming, W.E. (1986) *Out of the Crisis*, MIT Center for Advanced Engineering Study, Cambridge, Massachusetts.

Feigenbaum A.V. (1983) *Total Quality Control*, 3rd edn, McGraw-Hill Book Co., New York.

Ishikawa, K. (1976) *Guide to Quality Control*, Asian Productivity Organisation, Tokyo.

Ishikawa, K. (1985) *What is Total Quality Control? – the Japanese Way* Prentice-Hall, Englewood Cliffs, New Jersey.

Juran J.M. (1988) *Juran on Planning for Quality*, Free Press.

Juran, J.M. and Gryna, F.M. (1980) *Quality Planning and Analysis*, 2nd edn, McGraw-Hill Book Co., New York.

Koch, H.C.H. (1991a) Quality of care and service. *Managing Service Quality*, **July**, 1–5.

Koch, H.C.H. (1991b) Obstacles to total quality in health care. *International Journal of Health Care Quality Assurance*, **4**(3), 30–2.

Koch H.C.H. and Chapman, E.H. (1991) Planning for high quality care. *International Journal of Health Care Quality Assurance*, **4**(6), 10–18.

Oakland, J.S. (1986) *Statistical Process Control*, Heinemann, London.

Oakland, J.S. (1989) *Total Quality Management*, Heinemann, London.

Shewhart, W.A. (1931) *The Economic Control of Quality of Manufactured Products*, Van Nostrand,

Shingo, S. (1986) *Zero Quality Control: Source Inspection and the Poka-Yoke System* Productivity Press, Stamford, Connecticutt.

Taguchi, G. (1979) *Introduction to Off-Line Quality Control*, Central Japan Quality Control Association, Magaya, Japan.

Taguchi, G. (1981) *On-line Quality Control During Production*, Japanese Standards Association, Tokyo.

Wilson, C.R.M. (1987) *Hospital-wide Quality Assurance: Models for implementation and development*, W.B. Saunders, Ontario.

A case study of the implementation of Total Quality Management in an NHS setting

Following the identification of the roles and responsibilities at the most senior level in the organization, the next stage is to establish the functional units whose role is to plan the implementation of the quality improvement process at a local level. The actions necessary to achieve this aim are outlined below. The steps that follow are the practical aspects of implementation and we have discussed them in the order in which we tackled them, rather than in strict numerical order.

THE IMPLEMENTATION OF THE CROSBY APPROACH TO TOTAL QUALITY MANAGEMENT

The application of Crosby's 14 steps in practice is explored based on the experiences of one QIT. This team was responsible for a General Hospital with approximately 160 beds, offering a broad range of services to the local population, including acute medical and surgical beds, rehabilitation wards, casualty and outpatients. Staffing levels were approximately 400 whole time equivalents. Although significantly smaller than most general hospitals, it offered a microcosm of many of the functional units into which larger hospitals are divided, in that within it were a wide range of professional disciplines and different services. It was managed as a discrete unit, although it was ultimately accountable to a body of management elsewhere.

As such, many of the practical aspects used as part of the implementation process could be applied in a larger hospital, in the presence of extra co-ordination via a structure such as that outlined in Figure 6.5.

In terms of the structural diagram in Figure 6.5. the quality improvement team used in the case study is shown as QIT 1. It is accountable to the steering committee, and the Chair has access to this committee via the structural framework devised for implementation. The other QITs are on a separate, larger site; all within one hospital.

STEP 2: QUALITY IMPROVEMENT TEAM

Purpose: To run the quality improvement process.

The QIT is the group of staff who are given the responsibility of running the quality improvement process. Based on our experiences, the following guide-lines are recommended when selecting the appropriate individuals for the team and running the Quality Improvement Process:

Action 1

Senior management, in conjunction with heads of department and senior members of the professions need to identify all the individual staff who fall under their sphere of responsibility. In this case, it meant everyone employed at the hospital.

This is important, because ideally, the quality improvement team should consist of a broad cross-section of the staff it is supposed to represent.

Action 2

The QIT members are selected on the basis of fulfilling one or more of the following criteria:

- They are a member of senior management, whose support is crucial. On this basis, the Unit General Manager, Director of Nursing Services and the two Clinical Managers became QIT members.
- They are a head of department or senior member of a professional group that represents a significant proportion of staff employed by the hospital (or, in a larger hospital, a unit). On this basis, the Consultant Physician, Acting Superintendent Physiotherapist, Catering Manager, Operational Services

Manager and Medical Records Manager all became QIT members. At a later date, following a management restructuring, the Clinical Director also joined the QIT.

- They have a specific skill or expertise that is useful to the team. On this basis the TQM project co-ordinator and Acting Senior Nurse for Service Development (which included a responsibility for quality assurance and the nursing workload dependency system) became QIT members.

The rationale for selecting such a seemingly top-heavy group was that it is essential that the QIT has authority to act, i.e. that decisions can be taken within the meetings without needing to be approved by more senior managers at a later date. It was also essential that these key individuals are involved in, and committed to, the process as they are in the key positions to be able to cascade the quality improvement process throughout the organization. Resistance at this level could potentially undermine the whole implementation process. Finally, it was a way of demonstrating to staff that this process was sufficiently important for these individuals to devote a significant amount of their time to it.

Three months into the process, the QIT felt that more 'grassroots' input would be useful to help with the implementation process, as at this stage the Team was heavily involved in Step 5 (quality awareness). Two Ward Sisters and a Staff Nurse who had undergone the educational course also joined the team. The Sisters adapted well to their new role; the staff nurse experienced difficulties in fulfilling some of the roles and responsibilities of a QIT member, in spite of her initial enthusiasm. A key factor for this was in her lack of hierarchical authority to implement QIT decisions back in her area. This reinforced the need to retain this as one of the selection criteria for QIT members. Provision for grassroots staff to access the quality improvement process is made through some of Crosby's other steps.

Action 3

The QIT members need to undertake the relevant education to equip them with knowledge needed to implement and manage the quality improvement process. Details of this are given under Step 8 (employee education).

Action 4

The Terms of Reference need to be agreed between the QIT and the Steering Committee.

Action 5

The roles and responsibilities of individual QIT members need to be determined. This was done by having a facilitated 'QIT start-up day'. In practice, we found we needed a significant amount of time set aside to give the QIT a clear sense of purpose and direction. Participants generally felt it was helpful to have a facilitator with extensive experience in this approach offering support and advice, as many were unsure of what was required in the beginning, and concerned at the logistics of how to tackle such a large project.

Responsibilities of QIT members

QIT members had two key areas of responsibility. These were:

- To be the link person between the QIT and an allocated group of employees, external customers and suppliers (e.g. the ambulance service, General Practitioners, Community Health Councils, etc.). The hospital employees were divided up equally and logically between all QIT members. It was decided that managers for certain areas would always be the link person for their own staff. Very small staff groups, such as Occupational Therapy, were given a link person who commonly had communications with them, in this case, the Physiotherapist on the QIT; the Consultant Physician acted as the link person for all the medical staff. Every employee therefore had a QIT member to represent their interests. The communication was two-way, with information on QIT progress and decisions being passed on to staff by the members and staff feeding back their opinions and problems via the QIT member. Much effort was put into informing staff of these new arrangements (as described in Step 5 (quality awareness)).
- To be a 'step sponsor' for one of the 14 steps. The steps were allocated to the individual QIT members on the start-up day. This was done as fairly as possible, with members agreeing

to take on the sponsorship. The step sponsor is responsible for planning and co-ordinating this particular step. The selection of step sponsors was found to be important for two reasons: first, it cut down enormously the amount of planning and discussion on each step in meeting time. Each step sponsor would draw up an action plan for the step, circulate it to the team a week prior to the meeting, and make a 5-minute presentation at the next meeting. QIT members then had the opportunity to make further recommendations or alterations to the plan before approving it. This was much more effective than the whole team planning each step from scratch. It was then the responsibility of the link person to ensure that actions regarding this step were completed in their area. For example, if the step sponsor for education identified that 20 staff from each area would be allocated a place on a course in the next 3 months, it was the responsibility of the link person to ensure that 20 of their staff attended. Each step sponsor would report regularly to the QIT on progress and difficulties made with implementing their step. Again, this cut down on meeting time, as it prevented the necessity of each link person to report on the progress of all the steps in their specific area.

Second, it generated an action-oriented approach to the QIT meetings. Many of us had expressed reservations that we already spent too much time in meetings, and were anxious this should not become a group that sat around debating the philosophical points of quality. This was further enhanced by the use of the meeting techniques outlined below. It also ensured that none of the steps were overlooked, and that they were reviewed constantly.

Another advantage of adopting this approach was that it placed the onus for actions very firmly with specific individuals, and the workload was shared out equally. This was in contrast to many other meetings we attended, where some members contributed significantly less than others in forwarding the various committees' objectives.

There were two other roles to be assigned, those of Chair and Administrator. Both were selected by the QIT itself, which was felt to be important.

The role and responsibilities of Chair included chairing all the

meetings, using the techniques identified as important for
effective management of meetings through the educational
courses. It also involved representing the QIT via the steering
group. The QIT selected the Consultant Physician as the Chair.
This worked extremely well, both because of the skills of the
individual concerned and because it secured the active involvement of the medical staff; something many other TQM pilot
sites appeared to have difficulty doing.

The role of Administrator was more wide-ranging than that
of the traditional meeting secretary. This individual should have
considerable expertise in the quality improvement process and
should be able to act as an adviser to step sponsors in planning
their steps; the Quality Co-ordinator was selected for this role.

Action 6

Create a set of clearly agreed requirements for QIT meetings.

We were conscious that it was important that QIT team
members were seen to practise what we preached with regard
to 'getting it right the first time', and that the meetings were an
example of this. Drawing on the techniques learned from the
educational materials, the following requirements were found to
be useful. It was agreed to meet once a week for 1 hour:

- All meetings will start and finish on time.
- Timed agendas and relevant papers will be circulated to all
  members 1 week prior to the meeting.
- Agenda times will be adhered to.
- With the exception of annual leave and sickness, members
  will attend all meetings.
- Minutes from the meeting will be distributed to all members
  within 24 hours.
- All action assignments will be marked with a name and
  completion date in the minutes, and reviewed by the
  chairman as a weekly agenda item.
- QIT members will inform the administrator of any errors in
  minutes within 24 hours of receipt. Corrections will be circulated prior to the following meeting.

These may seem rather draconian, but the important factor in
meeting these requirements was that everyone had agreed
them.

Most of the team were frustrated by other meetings they attended that started late and ran way over time, had poorly thought-out agendas (or no agenda at all) with one item taking up the whole meeting time, a pile of essential papers being circulated in the same meeting as a decision on their content was expected, key members not turning up to meetings or sending apologies and then spending the subsequent meeting disagreeing with all the decisions agreed at the meeting they had missed, minutes from the previous meeting not distributed or circulated in the next meeting for approval, some individuals taking up most of the meeting time by arguing over the accuracy of previous minutes and action assignments not documented or completed.

In practice, these new guidelines proved effective. An audit was established to examine if these were conformed with and within 4 weeks the score had altered from one of 45% to one of 100% on all items. It was interesting to note the change of attitudes over this time. Initially, many were sceptical that these could be met. Once it was agreed that these were things the team was serious about, and they were seen to be achievable, everyone worked hard to meet the requirements.

For example, circulating the minutes within 24 hours may seem an impossible achievement. In practice, it was agreed that the minutes should be a brief factual reference of decisions taken, with actions arising marked as specified. They did not necessarily need typing, providing they were legible. This made it possible to meet the requirement.

Having established the team, the first 18 months of work was concentrated on the introduction of eight of the 14 steps, all of which needed to be considered in relation to each other. For example, there is little point setting target dates for staff to start measuring work processes or establishing groups to solve problems if they have not completed the relevant educational course to equip them with the skills to do this.

General learning points concerning co-ordinating these first eight steps of the Crosby approach are discussed at the end of this chapter.

In practice, the establishment of a team of this kind was found to be an extremely effective way of managing a project of this scale. It was felt to be completely unrealistic to expect one individual with a 'Quality' remit to their job to undertake this

on their own. Moreover, by encouraging local ownership of the
process and involving key individuals, many of the factors
important to effective change management were incorporated.
Once established, it offers potential as a useful vehicle for
implementing other associated projects, for example, resource
management or the contracting process. It was also found to be
a useful method for breaking down interdepartmental and professional barriers.

This is not to say there were not some difficulties. Initially
there were reservations as to the effectiveness of adopting this
approach. Some people were put off by the amount of 'jargon',
although this was largely overcome once the education was
completed. Others were sceptical of the motives for adopting
such an approach, as its implementation coincided with that of
applying for self-governing status. A general comment was that
it seemed a lengthy way of solving problems that could be
resolved by individuals 'just chatting' about them. However, it
was generally conceded that, although this seemed logical, it
was not something that happened as a matter of routine. This
was highlighted by the significant number of ongoing problems
within the organization that had been resistant to this approach.
Some individuals were more enthusiastic and supportive of the
process than others but, none the less, every member made an
active contribution. As the process progressed, visible improvements started to occur and the support for this approach
increased.

STEP 1: MANAGEMENT COMMITMENT

Purpose: To make it clear where management stands on quality.

The initial activity involved in this step was the drafting and
agreement of a quality policy. This was important for two
reasons. First, it created a debate at the most senior level in the
organization regarding their views on the quality standard for
the service they were managing. It also created the opportunity
for them to discuss this issue with their staff.

Second, it had to be followed by clear management action to
support the policy. Staff are quick to pick up on management
actions that undermine such policies.

Crosby (1979, p. 176) defines the policy as 'The state of mind held by the company personnel concerning how well they must do their jobs.'

It therefore needs to be short enough to remember, clear enough for all staff to understand and unambiguous. These were criteria the team found it very hard to fulfil. Writing the policy so early in the project meant many of us were still shackled by the traditions of the old culture. The sort of policy recommended by Crosby is 'We will provide error-free services, on time and within cost.' Many were anxious at the implications of adopting such a policy and displaying it publicly throughout the hospital. There was a concern that it might render us legally liable to comply with such a promise. The difficulty in being less definitive is that lots of 'weasel words' creep into the policy, making it ambiguous. For example 'We will endeavour to provide an error-free service, most of the time, and as close to our budget limits as possible.'

The other difficulty is that many staff confused the idea of a quality policy with that of all the other 'trendy' organizational statements that seem to be creeping into the NHS 'management-speak', for example, 'visions', 'mission statements' and 'philosophies', and were trying to compose these, rather than a quality policy.

Once the policy has been agreed, the question on how to communicate it with staff was raised. It was agreed that it should be printed on posters, signed by senior management and be displayed throughout the hospital. Key learning points were:

- It should not be distributed until the quality improvement process is well underway. Displaying it too soon means the initial impact is lost and it is viewed with cynicism.
- It should be ready prior to the educational courses being commenced with staff. Course facilitators found it a useful way of starting the process of convincing staff that management was really serious in its commitment to the quality improvement process (a fact that some staff were extremely sceptical about).
- It needs to be launched in conjunction with other activities that demonstrate to staff that the quality policy is not just words but is about positive actions to improve. They needed to appreciate that 'something different' was happening.

The launching of the quality policy was planned as part of Step 5 (quality awareness), and is outlined below.

Once the policy has been launched, staff invariably scrutinize management actions and behaviour and are quick to point out any dichotomy between the two. As part of the educational courses, managers list actions that they can undertake personally to demonstrate their commitment to quality to their staff.

Management actions to demonstrate commitment

These actions included:

- *Agreeing requirements with their customers and suppliers, and then meeting these every time.* This proved an effective method both for improving professional relationships; and identifying and resolving problems.
- *Undertaking the educational courses and meeting all the requirements for these.* This was important, because if managers were seen to miss sessions, or not complete action assignments from the workshops, it implied to staff they were not genuinely committed to the quality improvement process. It also put the facilitator in a difficult position, as staff would argue that they should not be expected to fulfil the course requirements either.
- *Talking to staff about their problems with work processes, and empowering them to solve them.* This was found to be much more effective than trying to solve them for them. It meant setting time aside for 'management by walking about,' and observing first-hand the difficulties staff encountered. Initially, managers were concerned about the amount of time they would have to devote to the quality improvement process. When asked how much time they could afford to devote to it, many stated they would be pushed to give 5%. As the project progressed it was realized it was necessary to devote 100% of their time to it. Everything they did in their daily work needed to be done in a 'quality' way, and meet the requirements right the first time; from answering the telephone to compiling a report. In practice, by doing this, more management time was made available because less time was spent on fire-fighting or re-work.
- *Attending awareness sessions, at times outside 'office hours'.*

- *Making resources available.* It was felt to be important to allocate funds to areas where finance was found to be the final barrier to effecting a solution to an ongoing problem. Lack of such support had the potential for staff quickly becoming disillusioned, and did not believe management was seriously committed. A key factor here was honesty. If a large investment of cash is needed and is unavailable, this needs to be explained, but with the manager exploring temporary solutions and agreeing to fund it in the future budget. For example, one ward identified it required new mattresses for all the beds. This was not possible in the current financial year. Funding was made available for a proportion of these, with a commitment to start a yearly mattress replacement programme. In the interim period, those that were condemned were replaced by other mattresses from elsewhere in the hospital, which, although not new, were still functional.

  It was our experience that the problems that could only be resolved by a financial solution were in the minority. The majority were reliant on improved communication and more effective use of current resources by improving work processes.

  It is also essential to ensure adequate funding for the initial training and materials. It was a major set-back when external funding for this project was ceased after 2 years, when there had been an expectation that it was for three. The staff, course facilitators and quality improvement team were extremely demoralized by this, and resultant modifications to the project plan were perceived by some staff as lack of management commitment to the quality improvement process.

The QIT also initiated a communication survey, based on a questionnaire circulated to staff to ascertain their views on the way the hospital was managed. Following data collection and analysis, workshops were held with staff to discuss results and invite their suggestions on how to act on problems identified. A list of management actions was drawn up, circulated and undertaken.

This step was one of the most difficult to draw up plans for, because it is largely reliant on senior management and professionals ensuring their behaviour is congruent with the written exhortations in the quality policy. However, peer support and the use of measurement were both useful in commencing this change. Such changes were slow and impossible to measure objectively, but as many of us internalized the concepts explained in the education, it was a common observation that there were changes in both attitude and behaviour.

STEP 5: QUALITY AWARENESS

Purpose: To provide a method of raising the personal concern felt by all employees toward the conformance of the product or service and the quality reputation of the hospital.

The process of raising staff consciousness on quality issues, promoting the vital contribution that all individuals had to offer in the quality improvement process and demonstrating how this could be achieved was a key objective of Step 8 (employee education). This was also reinforced through many of the other steps.

The QIT decided to tackle the awareness step fairly early in the planning stage, as there had been some publicity in the local press about our selection as a pilot site for total quality management, and staff were starting to question what this would involve.

The initial decisions that had to be taken were on what and when to communicate with staff. It was agreed the information needed to be presented clearly and to have some kind of local flavour to it. There was also concern that previous attempts at communicating information through distributing leaflets had not been particularly effective, and it was felt this was due to the impersonal nature of such an approach. The QIT was keen to enter into dialogue with staff and provide a forum that allowed them to ask questions and voice their concerns. It was felt this was another way in which management could demonstrate its commitment to the quality improvement process.

The timing of the initial communications was also important. It was agreed this should not happen immediately because the team had not yet drawn up the implementation plan for the 14 steps, and it was felt that clear statements needed to be made on how this plan would affect individuals. Eventually, a date 4 months into the process was selected. This had the advantage that all the team members would have completed their educational course and would therefore be more knowledgeable about the tools and techniques when questioned by staff. The planning process for all the steps would be completed well before this date, and it also allowed sufficient time to prepare the supporting literature and make adequate preparations to ensure that we got this exercise 'right first time'.

In view of the large numbers of staff that needed to be involved in this exercise, coupled with the problem of reaching the shift workers, it was decided a good way to meet the objective of enabling all staff to participate was to hold an 'awareness week'.

A number of sessions were arranged throughout the week, rotating between breakfast, lunch, tea and supper times, which meant that all shift workers had a slot occurring at least twice that week which they could attend. The format agreed for each 45-minute session was:

- An introduction and welcome from a senior member of management staff.
- A video 'starring' the Chair of the QIT, explaining the potential benefits of the quality improvement to staff and the importance of everyone's role.
- An exhibition consisting of poster presentations by each of the step sponsors explaining the plans for their step. This would enable staff to walk round and discuss these with individuals, enabling those who felt unable to ask questions in front of 30 or 40 other participants to do so on an individual basis.
- A short 'Crosby' video of an American Hospital, interviewing staff who were 2 years into the quality improvement process, explaining what was involved, and what had been achieved.

In view of the amount of information available to staff, it was felt to be important to give them a summary of the key points presented in these 45-minute sessions. A considerable amount of work went into designing a folder, which was handed to staff personally when arriving at the session. Learning from previous experience, the QIT avoided glossy pamphlets with photographs of members beaming forth from the pages and cheap, photocopied, poorly presented materials. Staff tended to be critical of the former, and viewed it as a waste of money that could be better spent elsewhere; and of the latter because it was seen as being 'done on the cheap'. The appropriate combination was felt to be in the form of a printed A3-sized folder; folded so that a cartoon of the distinctive hospital main doors opened out to show the information inside, with the caption 'Opening the door to quality' underneath. On the inside two leaves were the four absolutes of quality, and the quality policy. In the centre was the logo the QIT had designed with the slogan 'Total Quality Improvement: Putting the "U" in quality'. This had been arrived at after a brain-storming session, which had ruled out; 'Putting the "Y" in quality'; and 'Knocking the "L" out of quality'! Coming up with a slogan was felt to be a good way of getting the essence of the quality improvement programme across in a short, snappy, phrase. The '"U" in quality' stressed that this process was aimed at everyone, whether 'you' are the patient receiving a better service or the staff providing this. None the less, it was something that was alien to many of us and, in the beginning, many felt self-conscious about coming up with ideas.

The folder held information on what the quality improvement process involved and why it was important to the hospital. On the reverse of the folder were cartoons of all the QIT members; with the staff groups they represented on the team printed underneath. This 'lightened up' the message and gave it a local flavour. In the event, staff received the folder with interest, and found it helpful. We also seemed to have hit the right balance between it looking as though it was being done on the cheap and being a waste of money; at £80 for 400 folders we could hardly be accused of wanton extravagance.

The poster exhibition also featured cartoons from a local artist, with the accompanying text printed by the graphics department. This kept costs down, although the exhibition itself was clear, eye-catching and professionally displayed.

The Chair made an introductory video for the session, explaining why the hospital was embarking on this process. This was useful for the sessions, as clinical commitments meant he could not attend them all, and it ensured staff all got the same information.

The QIT debated how best to ensure a good attendance at the session throughout the awareness week. In view of the fact it was intended to demonstrate commitment to the new culture, many felt it would be inappropriate to 'instruct' staff to come. It was agreed all QIT members would approach their staff groups, tell them a little about the sessions and invite them to sign up to attend one on the quality notice board, which was placed in a strategic position on the way into the staff dining room. Management also agreed to fund provision of food at all these sessions. The team would like to think this had only a marginal influence on the subsequent pleasing attendance rate, with 320 attenders at the sessions over the week; approximately two-thirds of the staff. At the request of others who had been unable to attend, the exhibition remained up for a further week to allow the remainder of the staff to attend.

A short questionnaire was distributed for staff to fill in at the end of the session. This showed that the staff had found all aspects of the session useful, rating the poster presentation as most useful, closely followed by the locally produced video. Although the majority felt the Crosby video of some use, many did not like the 'Americanisms'. It also showed that the majority of staff felt positive about the concepts of the quality improvement process. Some cynicism was expressed in the form of comments by staff as to the ability of senior management and professionals in being able to make it work. There were some individuals who felt the whole exercise to be a huge waste of time, but these represented less than 1% of respondents.

The overall conclusions drawn from the questionnaire results were that the awareness week had fulfilled its objectives, and had been successful. Another benefit was that it had been the first time that many individuals on the team had worked together in this way, and a good feeling of camaraderie built up over the week.

The second stage in planning this step was in maintaining the initial momentum, and ensuring that the quality improvement process was given a continually high profile. This was achieved in the following ways:

- By continually updating the quality notice board. This included displaying lists of staff attending courses, measurements currently being made in different departments and results so far and details of problem-solving activities.
- By QIT members keeping their staff groups informed of developments.

- By printing articles written by staff about their quality improvement activities arising from the educational courses in the hospital newspaper.
- By planning the zero defects day (outlined as Step 9). This served to focus the efforts of the team on ensuring that effective communication occurred with staff. The approaches adopted above were an innovation, in that traditional approaches such as meetings and memorandums tended to be the norm.

A lesson learned was that it is not just the efforts of a team working on a project of this kind that is important, effective communication of the impact it will have on those who will be affected by it must also be given equal priority. This was crucial when the quality improvement process was cascaded throughout the hospital because if staff had a pre-conceived negative view, they were unlikely to become actively involved.

STEP 8: EMPLOYEE EDUCATION

Purpose: To define the type of education all individuals need in order to actively carry out their role in the quality improvement process.

The Crosby system offers a variety of educational courses aimed at meeting the educational needs of all the individuals within the organization. Although this case study examines only one specific approach, there are some generic guidelines learned from our experiences that can be extended to others wishing to establish TQM within an organization.

First, the educational needs will differ for different levels of the organization, and this is determined by the role taken in relation to the quality improvement process. These fall into the broad categories outlined below.

An executive-level course

This is required to focus on the role of those at executive level, and the actions needed to lead the quality improvement process in their organization. The course should incorporate the writing of a quality policy, the implementation process (in this case study this was the 14 steps), the establishment of a structure for managing quality and the tools and techniques.

Quality improvement for managers

There is a need for a course aimed at QIT members. This will need to outline the implementation process in detail to prepare team members for their new role. The workshops in the course used at the hospital in this case study facilitated consideration on adopting and implementing these steps at a local level. The final workshop involved drawing up an implementation plan for all 14 steps for the first year.

Quality education for the individual

It was identified that there was a need for a comprehensive course aimed at senior individuals within the hospital, who were a vital component in implementation of the quality improvement process.

The course used by the hospital in the case study included the four absolutes, the use of the process model work sheet, measurement, calculating the cost of quality, teamwork and problem-solving techniques; in essence, all the tools and techniques that will help individuals understand and manage their work processes. Individuals were given action assignments that enabled them to introduce these in their workplace.

Quality education for the work group

To start the process of resolving work-based problems, teams of staff need to work together. This process can be introduced through mixed educational sessions aimed at work groups. Such courses need to cover the basic tools and techniques, which (in the case study) the group apply in their workplace and return to the next session with the results for discussion.

Introductory course

To fit in with the concept of TQM, all staff should be involved in the educational sessions. For some, this will require a basic introduction to the concepts of quality. There is therefore a need for a less intensive course than for those with the different roles and responsibilities above. Such courses are also useful as part of the staff induction process.

Cascading the education through the organization

It is the role of the quality manager to commence the whole process of education, although this responsibility is delegated to the QITs once they are established. The logistics of planning an educational initiative that involves everyone in the organization involved significant time and effort. From our experiences, the following approach is recommended.

- *Those at the top of the organization must attend the appropriate courses first.* This is important, as without detailed knowledge of the implementation framework and the tools and techniques, it is difficult to lead the quality improvement process in the organization. It also gives the opportunity to review the educational packages and ensure they are suitable for use within the organization, and demonstrates commitment to the process.
- *All QIT members should attend the appropriate educational courses.* This provides them with the knowledge needed to implement the process (in the case study, the 14 steps). This enables them to start functioning as a team from the outset. It also provides the team with the tools and techniques for individual participation in the quality improvement process. This prepares them for when their staff attend the courses, and come to them to discuss their activities and work processes.
- *The QIT should select at least one member (usually the Education Step Sponsor) to be a 'master trainer'.* They take responsibility for training a number of individuals within the organization to enable the courses to be cascaded to all levels. The Education Step Sponsor will need to develop a training plan for all the employees represented by the team. This process ensures that everyone attends the appropriate course.

Cascading the educational process at a local level

The QIT tackled this by attending the initial courses as a group, combined with three other staff members. This had the advantage of developing the team and enabling them to begin to develop a multidisciplinary approach to problem-solving. Having 'grass roots' representation also had the advantage of beginning to break down some of the hierarchical barriers. With hindsight it is recommended that a good mix of staff, in terms of position, as well as discipline, creates the most productive sessions. It enables all staff to appreciate the roles and difficulties of others, often for the first time.

After completion of the quality course aimed at the individual's role in the quality improvement process, it was agreed by the QIT that each member needed support from someone else from the area they were representing on the team, who had the same insight into managing the quality improvement process. The second course therefore consisted of nominees recommended by QIT members.

Due to a few 'misunderstandings' clear requirements were set for following courses regarding selection and attendance, which vastly improved the whole process:

- Each QIT member would discuss the course with individuals from their area, and offer the opportunity to attend.
- Nominations were sent to the Educational Step Sponsor, with any dates or time when the individual was unable to attend a course (for example, due to annual leave or a busy time in the area).
- The nominees were allocated a place on a course that matched availability, and these were returned to the QIT member who nominated them.
- It was the responsibility of the QIT member to ensure the individual was informed of course details, and to ensure attendance on the course.

This approach worked well for the following reasons. First, the Educational Step Sponsor has little hierarchical authority in areas that fall outside their normal managerial 'patch'. By placing the onus on the manager, it prevented the situation arising where staff were not given 'permission' to go. This put the responsibility for staff education firmly with the manager, rather than the Educational Step Sponsor.

Second, it was a clearly agreed requirement that places allocated to an area must be filled. This ensured that, if an individual was sick or absent, the manager would allocate the place to someone else. This prevented the frustrating situation of running under-attended courses.

Finally, it offered an effective way of ensuring staff and management communicated about the quality improvement process.

Staff knew the manager had also done the course, and were shown the educational materials. This approach was found to reduce the complication of staff turning up claiming they had been 'sent' by their manager, but didn't know why they were there.

It was agreed as part of the education step plan that each area should have a Local Quality Course Facilitator. This was seen as a good way of having resource people, spread throughout the hospital, to whom staff could go for help and advice. Therefore if the QIT member was unwilling or unable to become an instructor, it was important the 'support' person they nominated for the educational course was willing to fulfil this role. In practice, this did not quite work out as planned, due to a combination of staff leaving and some inappropriate nominations.

However, a lesson learned was the importance of not making assumptions about how specific individuals might receive the course, and who might make good instructors. In the event we were surprised by a number of individuals who proved to be excellent instructors, some of whom had skills that managers were previously unaware of.

Nominations for quality courses were sent to the Education Step Sponsor by the QIT members, and courses were planned using the new facilitators who had attended the preparatory trainers' course.

General conclusions regarding implementation of this step

In terms of sheer scale, the education step is the one that involves the greatest amount of work. This led to some serious questioning of the need for all the different courses, and whether it was worthwhile providing education for every employee.

Once the QIT became familiar with the course content, the need for the different courses was appreciated. The key factor in selecting staff for courses was to consider the role they played in the quality improvement process. Early difficulties arose because staff attended an inappropriate course. For example, some staff struggled with the quality education aimed at the individual; the reason being they were not in positions that required them to become involved in a managerial capacity, and another course would have been more appropriate. Some staff struggled with the technical elements in the work group course, but would have benefited from a simpler, shorter course, such as the introductory course. Interestingly, we estimated a much higher number as needing the work group course than recommended by the Crosby method. This is probably due to the fact that the levels of accountability are pushed much lower in the NHS than in industry. For example, Enrolled Nurses, although appearing low down in the hierarchical pecking order, have considerable responsibility in terms of making decisions about patient care.

The Crosby courses used by the hospital in the case study did provide a comprehensive insight into the concepts and tools and techniques. There were some criticisms of the courses, predominantly about the Americanisms, the industrial bias and the 'soap opera' style videos. To be fair to the company, they have subsequently rewritten a health service version and have produced English videos. Some staff found the courses too easy, and others found them too hard. With hindsight, this was partly due to bad planning, and to some staff attending the wrong course. Medical staff in particular frequently commented it was 'long-winded', and it probably would have been more appropriate for them to do the shorter 'quality for the doctor' that has been developed recently.

The disadvantage of this is that the opportunity for them to mix in with the rest of the staff is lost; something that both Doctors and staff rated as valuable.

The course evaluations from the work groups' educational sessions were positive, and the QIT was encouraged by the high standard of project work produced by participants.

Other problems arose as a result of the way the educational process was cascaded throughout the organization. There was a management re-structuring 5 months into the start of the implementation of the quality improvement process. This meant that those at executive level did not attend the course until many of their subordinates had done so. There were some instances of staff approaching managers to discuss their action assignments, and the manager had not done the course. This situation is to be avoided at all costs, as it compromises both individuals.

Another difficulty arose as a result of some of the early attempts at educating potential QIT members. The initial consultancy firm selected by the steering group, used (unbeknown at the time) a 'Crosby-style' approach, although did not use their training materials. This meant that instead of the 4-day quality improvement process course for QIT members, a 2-day course was run on site. Although providing an insight into some of the concepts of TQM, it was not until four staff attended the Crosby quality improvement process course at the Crosby Quality College, that the limitations of the 2-day version were realized. The main problem was that too little time was spent on the 14 steps, or on the practicalities of implementation, which created difficulties for those expected to fulfil this role. By the time the decision to switch to the wholesale Crosby approach was taken, the next stage of the educational cascade had begun. Hence the majority of original QITs did not have any members who had completed the 'proper' Crosby course. The QIT mentioned in the case study was fortunate in that three of its members had attended the 4-day course, and it was agreed that this was beneficial both for these individuals and to the team, in terms of their increased knowledge on how to manage the implementation.

For these reasons it is impossible to draw general conclusions about the success or failure of the Crosby educational materials, as two of the essential elements advocated – implementation cascaded from the top of the organization and the use of the course designed specifically to enable the QIT to function effectively – were never realized.

What did become apparent to the QIT members cited in the case study was that, in spite of the difficulties of co-ordinating such an educational exercise, it was a crucial part in beginning the culture change previously mentioned. For many staff, it was the first time they had ever had the opportunity to contribute to the organization in this way. As one member of staff said 'I've worked here for 20 years, and it's the first time any one has asked my opinion on anything'.

The 'common language' used in the courses, combined with the tools and techniques taught, enabled staff to work with their peers at improving the work processes in which they were involved. It moved the focus away from the 'finger-pointing' culture of looking for people to blame when things went wrong to one that looked at identifying and agreeing requirements to ensure things went 'right first time'.

As more staff attended the courses, the purpose of the other 13 steps in supporting their efforts to improve became more apparent. Education alone is not enough, staff also require support and direction from a QIT through the setting of goals, a clear demonstration of management commitment, measurement charts and a system to enable problems identified through measurement to be solved, a framework to enable individual employees to communicate work problems to management, a continual awareness of their role in the quality improvement process and recognition of their efforts. These other steps, and the practicalities of implementation, will now be examined.

STEP 3: MEASUREMENT

Purpose: To provide a display of current and potential non-conformance problems in a manner that permits objective evaluation and corrective action.

Practicalities of implementation

The key responsibilities outlined by the step sponsor to ensure successful implementation of this step by the QIT members were:

- To pilot measurement charts and ensure they were printed in preparation for staff to use as part of the educational courses.
- To commence measurement of one of their own work processes as a method of demonstrating commitment to the importance of measurement to their staff.
- To act as a resource for staff to staff by helping them to commence measurement of their own work processes.
- To actively promote the use of measurement in their area.
- To make staff aware of measurement being conducted throughout the hospital, and actions arising as a result.

Staff were taught how to identify aspects of their work processes for measurement, and techniques for collecting and quantifying such data, as part of their education.

An advantage of the use of measurement was that it changed the terminology of the identification of problems from the subjective (which, under the traditional culture tended to blame specific individuals) to the objective (which described the problem in quantifiable terms that focused on deficiencies in the work process). For example, 'The linen room never supply us with enough linen at the weekend' becomes 'Over a 1-month period, sufficient linen to meet the ward's requirements for the weekend was not supplied for 53% of the time'. This is important in promoting meaningful dialogue between the individuals involved in the process (in this instance, the nurses, the porters, the linen staff and the laundry) as it focuses the attention on the problem, rather than jumping to conclusions about the cause. Further measurement may show that there is insufficient linen in circulation to meet the weekend demand, that the stocks ordered by nurses are insufficient or that there are insufficient porters on at the weekend to deliver the linen.

Staff were encouraged to display their measurement charts in the work area, which served as a focal point for discussion with staff and management, as well as identifying clearly the impact of methods being used in an attempt to solve the problem. There were exceptions to this rule if it was felt patients may misconstrue data presented, for example, the number of errors on a prescription chart, which referred to drugs not signed for and, in turn, to start and stop dates not completed, rather than to drug errors.

A number of key lessons were learned in implementing this step. These were as follows.

Guidelines when implementing measurement

Staff education
Staff education was essential in reducing the threatening nature of measurement. In areas where staff were asked to measure aspects of their work prior to attending the quality educational courses, this was treated with fear and mistrust.

Positive attitude to measurement
It was crucial for management to be positive about the use of measurement, even if this identified deficiencies in the service. Using the results of data collected in this way as a method of chastising staff for their performance was a short-cut to guaranteed failure of the whole quality improvement process, as it undermined the whole philosophy of the culture change it was attempting to achieve.

Full knowledge and co-operation

No measurement should be carried out on another department or profession without their knowledge and co-operation. There were initial concerns that this would skew the results, as it would be probable that extra effort would be made to ensure requirements were met if staff knew these were being measured. In practice, in the case of genuine failure of specific work processes, this was difficult to maintain over the extensive period that the data were being collected. The benefits of including other areas in this way were two-fold. First, it ensured that the data collection was done in a way that was accepted by those being measured as valid, and that the part of the process being measured was a reliable indicator of how the process was working. For example, a ward may be unhappy about the quality of the patients' meals. The nurses measure the number of 'errors' (such as patients receiving food they did not order, items missed from the plate etc.). They have a pre-conceived idea that this is due to inadequacies in the catering department. They present the 40% non-conformance rate of the catering staff as evidence of their 'failure'. The catering department has also been concerned about the problems with the same process. They use a different criterion and measure the number of incomplete or illegible menus that are returned to the kitchen. They present the 60% non-conformance rate to the nursing staff as evidence of their 'failure'. Here, measurement creates barriers between the departments. A more effective method is to convene a group of representative individuals from all the disciplines involved in the process and, using the tools and techniques such as the process model worksheet, look at ways in which they can work together as a team to improve the process. In this instance, measurement is used to identify deficiencies in the process, rather than in looking to assign blame to specific individuals.

By using the staff to measure their own work processes, with the specific objective of identifying an area in need of quality improvement, the data collected tended to be more accurate than under the traditional 'hit squad' style of quality assurance. For example, if staff know there is to be a health and safety check, they tend to tighten up on all the factors they know will be audited and the data collected do not necessarily present a true picture of normal practice.

Conversely, a member of staff who is concerned about the severe lack of storage space on the ward, may choose to audit the number of occasions when items were found to be blocking the fire escapes. It is probable that the number of instances would not reflect the findings of the health and safety check. This is because the presence of the staff member on the ward would not be seen as intrusive, and it is more difficult to fool staff who are based permanently on the ward in this way. The people who understand where the non-conformances commonly arise are those most closely involved in the work process.

Staff involvement

The staff themselves should determine which aspects of the work process to measure. Staff who selected an area of measurement because it was something that was causing them a lot of problems at work produced markedly more accurate and better presented data than a minority staff who had been instructed to measure things in which they had little interest. The course facilitators were able to recommend appropriate ways of collecting data once the staff had selected the work process which they felt required improving.

Staff were encouraged to pick one, or a maximum of two things to measure, using the general guide-lines outlined above. They were supported by their course facilitator and QIT member in carrying out their measurement. It was quickly identified that staff at all levels within the organization working in this way on a number of small-scale projects could, collectively, have a significant impact on improving the service. There were instances where staff measured processes that were perceived by them to be a problem, yet measurement proved that this was not the case. This was in itself important, as some areas had been branded with the label of not meeting requirements, which (in some cases) was unwarranted. The types of requirements measured crossed a huge range in both diversity and scale. Examples include:

- Waiting time for outpatient clinics.
- Consultants not arriving on time to start clinics.
- Incorrectly addressed mail.

- Number of incorrectly completed forms.
- Meetings starting and finishing on time.
- Requests for directory enquiries via switchboard.
- Wheelchairs not conforming to requirements.
- Patients' personal laundry returned to wrong ward.
- Wasted items in CSSD packs.
- Nursing time spent on clerical duties.
- Menus returned to kitchen by required time.
- Inappropriate GP referrals to physiotherapist.
- Medical records lost or mislaid.
- Urgent requests met on time.

The results from such measurements gave a clear indication of the scale of the problem and also provided a useful baseline against which to compare the impact of actions subsequently taken to resolve the problem. The measurements themselves often provided the staff with essential information needed to present their case for the need for improvement to occur. For example, it was found that over half of the hospital wheelchairs did not conform to requirements (i.e. tyres pumped up, all footrests and armrests present and functioning, wheelchairs clean and stored in the correct areas). This presented a powerful case for the need to purchase some new wheelchairs, and for staff to agree requirements on maintaining them in good working order. Under a traditional hierarchical culture, many staff would have resented an extra task such as wheelchair maintenance being added to their job. In this instance, because the staff themselves had identified that they were wasting a significant amount of their time 'fixing' wheelchairs and that there was a risk to patients, and because they had identified the solution for themselves, the process could be improved. A crucial part in this was in management accepting this measurement and purchasing some new wheelchairs as part of the solution.

The final item on the list posed some interesting debates, as it was realized that no one had ever established a definition of 'urgent'. Hence, portering staff were constantly told a job was 'urgent'. In practice, only a proportion of these required immediate attention, for many others a clear requirement such as 'within 1 hour' or 'before midday', would enable them to plan their work more effectively.

General conclusions regarding the implementation of this step

The introduction of widespread, systematic measurement throughout the hospital is an essential part of quality management. There was also some sound theoretical underpinning in introducing it with the support of some of the other steps outlined in this approach. Returning to the theories of effective management of change in Chapter 4, measurement proved to be an extremely effective method of 'unfreezing' or helping staff to perceive the need for change. The fact that they 'owned' the data they were collecting was an important part of its being accepted as valid. The biggest obstacle to its introduction was in overcoming the mistrust of the way in which such data might be used. There was a strong initial suspicion that there was some hidden, ulterior motive on the behalf of management. It was therefore essential that staff believed in the commitment of management to the quality improvement process, and were convinced that measurement would not be used to their detriment.

Two other crucial steps in changing the culture to enable measurement on this scale to occur were the education of all staff and the establishment of a corrective action system. The education equipped everyone with the knowledge and skills needed to measure their work, as well as helping them to appreciate its benefits to them personally. It was essential that a corrective action system existed to resolve the problems raised through measurement. In the event of staff being unable to solve these problems themselves, a mechanism was needed to ensure that it reached the level in the organization that could effect a solution. If nothing changed as a result of measurement, staff motivation to continue will diminish quickly. This step will now be explored.

STEP 6: CORRECTIVE ACTION

Purpose: To provide a systematic method of resolving forever the problems that are identified through other action steps.

Tackling this step fell into two broad categories. First, the education of all staff in the principles of problem solving, second, the development of an infrastructure that supported them in this process. This was necessary to ensure that problems that could not be resolved at a local level reached the appropriate level for action to occur. These two categories are outlined below.

The five-step problem-solving method

This technique involves five stages, which participants on the educational courses apply to their work-related problems.

Step 1: Define the situation

This step draws heavily on the measurement step. The situation that is causing the difficulty must be measured, both to establish the size of the problem and to enable it to be expressed in objective, rather than subjective, terms.

For example, medical photography may identify that 12 out of 24 pictures do not 'come out'. When asked to define this situation, typical answers include 'the camera was faulty', 'they weren't developed properly' or 'the photographer made a mistake with the exposure'. Such responses illustrate the traditional approach to problem solving we have identified in the Health Service. The definition of the Medical Photographer's problem is that '12 out of 24 pictures did not come out'. The other answers do not define the situation; they make assumptions as to the *cause* of the situation. In doing this, there is a danger that the assumption is incorrect, and therefore the subsequent action taken to resolve the perceived (rather than the actual) causes of the problem are ineffective.

Step 2: Fix

This stage involved introducing a temporary solution to the problem in order to enable the process to continue to function.

In practice, we found that this is the stage at which many of the organizational problems were. The hospital was full of evidence of 'quick fixes', which quickly became the norm. These included wheelchairs, cot sides and other equipment held together by strapping tape; an extra checking stage built into many processes, such as forms being checked and authorized by up to three different managers; over-ordering or overbooking in the expectation the process will not deliver as expected (for example, assuming a 25% non-attendance rate in outpatients and holding a month's worth of stock instead of the required 2 weeks' because of lack of confidence in the delivery system).

Step 3: Identify the root cause

This stage involved further measurement and analysis of the problem to ascertain the underlying cause. For example, the Medical Photographer may have the camera serviced or check on the stages of the development process to analyse what the root cause of the problem is.

Step 4: Take corrective action

This stage involved taking action to eliminate the root cause. For example, if the Medical Photographer finds that the development solutions are past the expiry date they should be discarded and new ones bought.

Step 5: Evaluate and follow up

The final stage involves the evaluation of the solution using further measurement to establish whether the problem has been resolved. In the above example, the Medical Photographer would inspect subsequent batches of photographs to ensure all 24 come out, and review this periodically to ensure the process is working properly.

The five-step problem-solving method enables individuals to solve problems related to their work processes. However, there will be occasions when they are unable to resolve these alone. A system to ensure they receive the appropriate support is necessary; this is described below.

Creating an infrastructure to co-ordinate and support problems

It is estimated that approximately 80% of problems identified can be solved at a local level. The remaining 20% require the

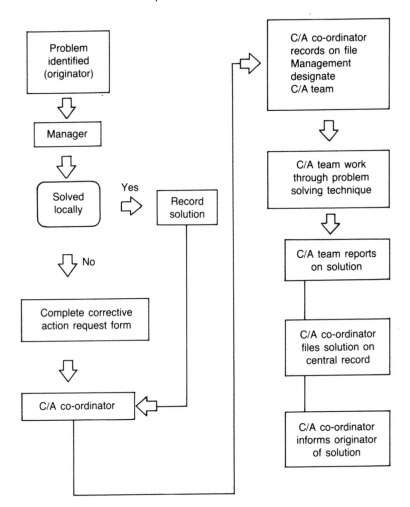

Figure 7.1 The corrective action system.

involvement of other individuals, either for the purpose of effecting a solution, or in order to release some funding (Crosby, 1991). In practice, we found this figure to be extremely accurate.

Based on our experiences, it is recommended that the planning and implementation of this step is tackled in the following way.

First, the Steering Group, in consultation with the Corrective

Action Step Sponsors from all the QIT's, designs and process-proves a corrective action system for use throughout the whole organization. This should be fully functional prior to the education of the staff. This is important, both so that the documentation supporting such a system can be introduced to course participants and to ensure that the system is ready to support staff immediately they require to use it. Confidence in management commitment fades quickly if significant efforts on behalf of staff are not met with the support promised. An example of a corrective action system is shown in Figure 7.1.

How the corrective action system works

In the event of a problem that requires actions outside the scope of the individual, the member of staff identifying the problem, and their QIT member, complete a 'corrective action form'. This has two benefits. First, it promotes dialogue on the problem, which can often be resolved by the manager and staff member as a result of this meeting alone. Second, it prevents misuse of the system by individuals who have not carried out the initial stages of problem-solving themselves (i.e. define the situation, fix and identify root cause) and are attempting to 'dump' the problem on their colleagues.

If the problem requires entry into the system, the QIT member will pass it on to the Corrective Action Step Sponsor, who will present it at the next QIT meeting. The role of the QIT is to discuss which individuals need to form a 'corrective action team' to resolve the problem. These should consist of the individuals who are closely involved in this work process, and able to contribute to an effective solution.

The corrective action team is then formed and uses the tools and techniques learnt as part of the quality educational courses to resolve the problem. The Corrective Action Team Leader communicates the progress of the team via the appropriate documentation, to the Corrective Action Step Sponsor. This is important, as once a large number of teams are established, there is a need to maintain a central focus on all the various projects. It also ensures that corrective action teams do not just sink without trace into oblivion.

If the team reaches a point where it does not have the necessary authority to act (although this should not be a problem if membership was considered carefully in the first instance) then the Corrective Action Step Sponsor raises the difficulty at QIT level, and the QIT will pass the information on the problem and progress to date to the appropriate manager for action and a progress report within a specified period of time.

When the problem is resolved, all the details are retained by the Corrective Action Step Sponsor as a central record, and the QIT member responsible for Step 12 (recognition) ensures that the efforts of the team are recognized in an appropriate way. The corrective action team is then disbanded.

General conclusions regarding the implementation and use of this step

The five-step method of problem-solving proved to be an extremely logical and useful tool, which was adopted quickly by staff. Although initially viewed by some as 'pure common sense', and subsequently unnecessary, the large numbers of unresolved problems that were identified as the quality improvement process was implemented were a clear indication that, in spite of some claims to the contrary, there was no systematic approach to solving problems within the hospital. These were traditionally tackled on an *ad hoc* basis, with no mechanism for monitoring and co-ordinating these efforts.

A crucial element in the successful implementation of this step is to establish culture that recognizes and values the contribution of all staff, and empowers all individuals within the organization to contribute actively to solving problems. This often involves delegation of responsibility, which can prove extremely threatening for some managers, who feel their position of authority is being undermined. It requires different skills from that of the traditional line manager, requiring the ability to empower staff and support and develop individuals to enable them to make their own contribution to the quality improvement process, rather than problem-solving remaining exclusively within the domain of management.

The corrective action system, as outlined in Figure 7.1, was initially viewed by the QIT as overly bureaucratic, cumbersome and too complicated. In the event, this step was not given high priority, and left until much later in the implementation process. Resistance to the system was exacerbated by the terminology used. 'Corrective action' sounded rather Draconian, and generated visions of leather-clad, whip-wielding individuals striding through the hospital corridors. Early attempts to re-name this step failed miserably, as this simply seemed to replace one type of jargon for another. In practice, most of the course facilitators referred to this step as 'problem solving'.

As the implementation of the quality improvement process progressed, four major problems became apparent. These were as follows:

- *Staff were working on problems that the QIT was completely unaware of.* This had profound implications when evaluating the impact of the quality improvement process, as there was no record of either the impact of these projects, or on identi-fied price of non-conformance that needed to be incorporated into Step 4 (the cost of quality). It also meant that work was being duplicated, and some areas were subject to extra-ordinary stresses, which led to friction between departments rather than building bridges, as intended. For example, large numbers of staff expressed an interest in working on projects requiring a considerable amount of input from the catering department. The QIT needed to intervene to ensure no further projects were started until the current corrective action teams were disbanded. The reasons were explained and accepted by staff, some of whom assisted individuals who had started work in this area, whilst others selected equally worthwhile projects.
- *If staff were unable to resolve problems at a local level, they had no mechanism for seeking help once all the normal channels were exhausted.* The difficulty here was the lack of a system to ensure that problems reached the level in the organization where someone could help. Typically, many projects were floundering because of lack of a decision from a senior-enough level to authorize a change in work processes. On other occasions, significantly large problems were not being resolved due to the inability of individuals to secure financial support needed to effect a solution.
- *The QIT digressed into a corrective action team.* For team members who thrived on solving difficult problems, the temptation to provide instant solutions was too great to resist. This was detrimental for two reasons. First, it detrac-

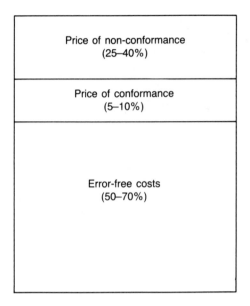

Figure 7.2 Cost of quality: a breakdown of expenditure (from Crosby, 1991).

ted from the real role of the QIT in managing the implementation of the 14 steps, and meant valuable meeting time was spent discussing a myriad of organizational problems. Second, it contravened the whole underlying philosophy of the culture change we were attempting to implement, in that we were imposing our solutions to problems within work processes that the staff involved in them were far more qualified to deal with. Furthermore, such imposed solutions bypassed all the essential mechanisms imperative in gaining staff ownership and acceptance of the required changes.

- *A number of problems that were common to the whole organization, and not unique to our QIT were identified.* This created the potential difficulty of ten QIT's working on the same problem with no central co-ordination.

These four problems threatened to reduce the quality improvement process to a series of uncoordinated quality initiatives. However, it was a useful learning experience, as it led to the appreciation of the need for the corrective action step, which offered a solution for the first three problems.

The fourth problem was resolved by forming a corrective action subcommittee, chaired by a senior member of the organization, and consisting of the Corrective Action Step Sponsors from all the QITs. The subcommittee's initial role was to establish an effective corrective action system that could be adopted uniformly throughout the organization. The role of this committee would later change to one of monitoring the large numbers of diverse projects, and co-ordinating the efforts of all the QITs. It also provided a forum for introducing problems that could not be resolved at QIT level, and needed raising at steering group or executive level.

A significant number of the problems raised through this step were found to be causing a significant financial cost to the organization. This will now be explored.

STEP 4: COST OF QUALITY

Purpose: To define the ingredients of the cost of quality and explain its use as a management tool.

The 'cost of quality' was an unfamiliar tool for those of us within the Health Service, although one that was relatively easy to grasp and utilize once the concepts had been explained as part of the educational courses. Put simply, the annual budget can be divided up as illustrated in Figure 7.2 (Crosby, 1991).

The price of conformance is the cost of doing business right the first time. For example, checking stock expiry dates in pharmacy, calibrating equipment, storing food at the correct temperature.

The price of non-conformance is the cost of not doing things right the first time. Hence every time a requirement is not met there is a knock-on cost in terms of time, money and human costs, from the set of medical notes going missing (causing extra work for the clerks) to the patient receiving the wrong operation. Often, the smaller errors are regarded as inevitable and are tolerated by staff and patients.

The error-free cost is the normal cost of doing business, for example heating, lighting, staffing, etc.

The advantages of calculating the price of non-conformance are:

- *It is an effective tool in directing management attention to a problem.* For example, dressing packs in the casualty department often have blunt scissors. This necessitates opening another pack, which is wasted. Staff measured these instances and calculated the cost of the wasted packs; it was £7,000 per year. To replace all the scissors would cost £400. Such information is useful when prioritizing expenditure.
- *It can act as a catalyst for problem solving.* For example, it was found in one area that 9% of patients coming for routine surgery either did not arrive or were cancelled as unfit for theatre. The cost to the hospital (calculated by adding the cost of admission, administration, and lost revenue) was £96,000 per annum. A multidisciplinary team was established to examine ways for reducing this problem.
- *It can redirect resources for more appropriate use.* For example, following the reduction in portering staff, an extra nurse was needed on the surgical ward to take patients to theatre. This had resulted in excessive over-time payments when theatre over-ran; it was calculated these would pay for a part-time porter. Furthermore, the nurse was then able to use her skills more appropriately.
- *It can act as a useful baseline measure.* This enables managers and problem-solving groups to compare the price of non-conformance from year to year and monitor progress.

Potential problems identified in using the tool

Some disadvantages were:

- Some managers may view it as a cost-cutting exercise.
- Staff may find it extremely threatening.

These problems can be avoided if cost of quality is introduced within a planned framework for implementing TQM. Managers and staff will therefore all have attended educational courses. It is most powerful and accurate when all levels within the organization use it.

Conducting the cost of Quality exercise

The collection of data on the price of non-conformance is divided into two phases. Phase 1 is the initial organizational exercise undertaken at the commencement of the quality improvement process, which is designed to give a very broad overview of the potential scope for improvement. This exercise can be repeated on an annual basis to monitor the impact of the quality improvement process. Phase 2 involves the collection of more specific data by those actually involved in the work processes, and the collation of such data to create a more accurate organizational cost of quality profile.

The phase 1 cost of quality exercise gathers data on the key areas where requirements are not being met the first time. It was commonly found that, for many work processes, there were no set requirements, particularly at interfaces between different departments or different professional boundaries. With the help of the unit accountant, a cost was then put on this data to estimate the overall price of non conformance.

This data was collected over a 2-day survey, during which a representative sample of a wide range of senior staff from all disciplines and areas, within the organization were interviewed.

Typical findings from a cost of Quality exercise

Studies carried out in a number of NHS units show similar problem areas arising.

Bed utilization problems

Examples typically include doctors spending a significant amount of time ringing round to find a bed for a patient, 'sleepers out' staying in hospital for longer than necessary, 'bed blocking' and acute beds used for 'social' admissions because of insufficient community back-up. Such findings are supported by a recent report by the Audit Commission, which estimated that the present level of activity in medicine could be provided by 58,000 beds, rather than the 85,000 currently in use (Audit Commission 1991).

Re-treatments

Prior to the introduction of medical audit there was little information on the extent of re-treatment of patients (either due to incorrect initial diagnosis or because of patient non-compliance). Also falling into this category are iatrogenic complications, with hospital-acquired infection and treatment of pressure sores costing the health service millions of pounds per year (Hibbs, 1988).

Work-flow problems

This is a knock-on effect of the interface problems outlined above. Examples include theatre teams waiting for up to 40 minutes for the porter to bring a patient, porters arriving to collect patients who are not ready and clinics running late. These problems are not the fault of the individual, but are due to unrealistic or unclear job requirements.

Firefighting

This is a common complaint from nursing and managerial staff. They seem to spend a large proportion of their time (up to 30%) repeatedly solving the same problems arising from work processes that are unable to meet service demands, or are not done right the first time. For example, forms filled in incorrectly, searching for lost items (ranging from medical notes to patients' false teeth!), trying to obtain laundry at weekends and what is commonly referred to as 'nipping' to other areas to deliver/collect things (e.g. drugs or equipment).

Wasted materials

In spite of the efficiency savings of recent years, there would still seem to be a large amount of wastage of materials. Examples include drugs expiring because of poor rotation and over-stocking, and poor stock management overall.

Unnecessary tests

Medical audit has, in many areas, identified a significant number of unnecessary or inappropriate tests.

Poorly run meetings

This is a common area identified by staff, i.e. that they start late, important people are not present (or others are present who get no value from the meeting), they do not produce positive actions and they over-run.

The results from the Phase 1 cost of quality exercise are fed back to senior management at the end of the second day. This was found to be an important part in helping senior management realize the potential benefits in embarking on quality improvement. Such improvement cannot occur under the traditional management culture outlined earlier. It requires a significant amount of resources both in time and money to reach the point where the cost of quality is reduced. Most of the authors with experience of this approach advocate between 3 and 5 years to reach the point where significant financial savings are seen as a by-product of the quality improvements that arise through this approach. It is important to stress that the costs that are reduced in this way are a beneficial consequence of the quality improvement process, rather than the underlying key objective. These benefits can only be realized by introducing a change in management culture, which needs to be supported by education, recognition and a firm management commitment.

General conclusions regarding the introduction of this step

There was little doubt that this tool was viewed as extremely threatening by the QIT. At the time of implementation there were simultaneous widespread changes in management structure as a result of the White Paper reforms, occurring against a backdrop of rumours about financial difficulties. The QIT accepted that such information could prove useful to them, but there were widespread concerns at all levels within the hospital regarding the way in which this information would be used. The primary concern was that staff would 'improve' themselves out of a job. Two factors were identified as important if the tool was to be accepted:

- That some of the savings made as a result of improvement should be made available to the QIT to plough back into the quality improvement process.
- That potential savings identified would not be subtracted from the budget allocation for the following year.

The second point was particularly important once the phase 1 cost of quality was completed. The data collected in phase 1 are intended to give a very general picture of areas that could benefit from improvement, rather than areas where budgets can be cut. Although some of the savings identified will fall back to the 'bottom line', there are also a significant number of others that cannot be realized in this way.

We likened it to our approach to shopping, when we may have a budget of £100 to spend on a dress. On spotting a 'bargain' that is reduced from £100 to £50, we spend the remaining £50 on a pair of shoes, also reduced from £100. We are delighted because we have 'saved' £100, even though the money is never liquidated. The important thing is that we get much better value for our money. Similarly, in the case of staff time wasted on dealing with work processes that do not work effectively, such as the example of the two whole time equivalent nurses walking backwards and forwards to Pharmacy, improving this process does not mean that two nurses are no longer needed. However, the proportion of all the nurses' time that went to make up the figure of two whole time equivalents can now be devoted to other, more appropriate, activities.

In practice, the majority of staff undertaking the work group educational course were far less sensitive about the use of the phase 2 cost of quality tool than had been previously imagined. It did prove to be a major factor in helping them to identify many of their processes that were not functioning well. As many commented 'We'd never considered how much time/money was wasted, we just considered it as inevitable'. They also found the calculation techniques taught as part of the course extremely useful in demonstrating to management the financial implications of deficiencies in work processes that required minor financial investment to correct.

For example, Medical Records did not have a paper shredder, and the £2,000 required to purchase one was not a high priority for the budget-holders. This necessitated clerks having to tear the records manually. Measurement calculating the average time spent by all the clerks tearing notes, when calculated on a *pro rata* basis, came to approximately £6,000 per annum. This did not mean the purchase of a shredder would mean the loss of a part-time member of staff due to time saved, but that the considerable back-log of work in this department could begin to be cleared as a result of extra time available. Having identified and realized savings in this way, most staff had no objection to these being publicized.

The other advantage of developing a phase 2 cost of quality, is that it is a way of illustrating the financial return on the initial investment made in staff training and solving problems. With hindsight, it would have been advantageous to complete the planning and implementation of this step far more thoroughly than was done in practice.

The figure identified as the 'cost of quality' was significantly high enough to cause grave reservations about expressing it in terms of cash, in case this was misconstrued in some quarters. Management was more comfortable to express the figure in terms of a percentage of the annual budget. Surveys of this kind conducted in the NHS show figures ranging from 23 to 30% of the total budget.

This may paint a depressing picture but, in fact, it is not significantly worse than many other organizations in both the public and private sectors. What it does illustrate is the scale of opportunity that exists if staff work positively together to solve these problems.

The benefits will not be realized through a conventional cost-cutting approach, with all its negative implications. The key is to empower the staff to talk in a constructive manner about the problems they have, and to give them the time and resources to tackle them systematically through a structured approach to quality improvement.

It is essential to recognize the efforts of staff who contribute in this way to the quality improvement process. Methods that can be used to achieve this are explored below.

STEP 12: RECOGNITION

Purpose: To appreciate those who participate.

The purpose statement for this step was an accurate phrasing of what many QIT members acknowledged was something that was lacking in the traditional NHS culture. The word 'appreciate' is used in the same context as when referring to art or antiques; it refers to adding value to something. There were widespread complaints from both ends of the hierarchy about being under valued and unappreciated. Many cited examples of extra efforts made, and the fact they were never thanked for these. Many managers acknowledged that they were so over-loaded with sorting out all the everyday problems, they spent more time expounding on what was wrong with the system than what was right with it. Although they acknowledged there were individuals who were reliable, hardworking and putting in extra effort, many felt unsure as to how to demonstrate their appreciation without seeming patronizing or insincere. They also felt unappreciated.

The QIT addressed this step by discussing with their staff groups what forms of recognition would be considered appropriate. The two key areas of enquiry were: (i) what sorts of actions required recognition; and (ii) how such actions could be acknowledged. The key recommendations presented to the team as a result of these discussions were as follows:

- That staff felt that actions that involved extra effort over and above their normal job role warranted recognition. Many commented that a simple 'Thank you' or occasional 'Well done' would be much appreciated. It was also felt those attending courses should receive some kind of recognition on successful completion.
- That staff felt the selection of individuals for recognition would have greater value if they were nominated by their colleagues rather than by management. Those nominated by management tended to be viewed in the same way as the 'teacher's pet' at school.
- There was a strong feeling that financial recognition for efforts was inappropriate. Although a minority felt that if their contribution saved the hospital millions of pounds they should receive a proportion; the majority stated they would prefer to see it re-invested in patient care. Many stated they would like to see some of it invested in their project or area.
- There was a strong feeling, particularly amongst QIT members that there needed to be a sum of money set aside specifically for the purpose of recognition. This was seen as an important way of demonstrating management commitment.

As a result of the discussions and planning, the following suggestions were implemented as part of this step:

- All staff who completed any of the educational courses received a certificate of attendance, signed by the Chief

Executive and presented by a QIT member, at the end of the course. Staff valued the certificate as something they could add to their curriculum vitae, and in spite of reservations about the presentation of these at the end of the course, the majority of staff appreciated this. The fact that senior members of staff had taken the trouble to attend the final session and take an interest in their projects did much to curb initial scepticism about the extent of management commitment. If many senior managers were honest, they were far more self-conscious about presenting these than those staff receiving them, which was perhaps a reason why this suggestion was not originally well supported.

- Each educational course chose to have a group photograph taken on completion, which was framed and displayed. These were received in good humour, and were a good illustration of the numbers of staff who had successfully completed these courses.

- Completed quality improvement projects, measurements being undertaken and other quality improvement efforts were displayed on the quality notice board with the names of those involved. This had two benefits: (i) it was a useful method of sharing ideas amongst staff, some of which were then implemented elsewhere; and (ii) it facilitated peer recognition, as many individuals were contacted by other staff for further information about their efforts. A number of these were also reproduced in more detail and printed in the hospital newspaper.

- There was a concerted effort on behalf of the QIT members to be more active in seeking out staff and praising them for their efforts. This was made much easier once the mechanisms for co-ordinating the corrective action step were established, as all QIT members were kept informed of the efforts of staff. It also included the acknowledgement within the QIT of the efforts made by its members both verbally, in terms of thanks from the Chair, and documented within the QIT meeting minutes.

- Approximately 3 months after completing the educational course, participants attended a 'follow up' session. The session was designed to be informal and was co-ordinated by one of the course facilitators. Each individual gave a brief summary of the process they had selected for improvement, the results from their measurement, and their progress in using the five-step problem-solving method. Each session was attended by at least two QIT members, who were responsible for feeding back the progress to the QIT. These sessions proved successful. First, staff were enormously supportive of the efforts of their peers, and gave them a great deal of encouragement. In instances where projects were experiencing set backs, many came in with offers of help, and it proved an effective way of breaking down professional and hierarchical barriers. Second, the fact that staff outnumbered the management present seemed to give them the confidence to identify areas in which they required more help and support. These comments were then raised at QIT level, with specific QIT members being actioned to help remove any 'road blocks' identified by staff. Actions taken were reported to the individual member of staff, as well as the QIT. All staff attending these days received a personal letter of thanks for their efforts, with confirmation in writing of any actions promised as a result.

- One year into the process, a conference was arranged with a lunchtime exhibition featuring poster presentations of all the project work completed by staff as part of the educational courses. Over 60 projects were submitted for presentation. This forum provided an excellent opportunity for senior management and peer colleagues to acknowledge the efforts of these staff. Two of the completed projects were selected for special recognition, and these staff were presented with a book token by the Chair of the Health Authority. These projects involved the establishment of a counselling service for women admitted for breast surgery by an Enrolled Nurse and a Registered Nurse, and the introduction of teaching sessions and a resource pack aimed at increasing staff knowledge on the system for ordering stores. This was the project of a member of the office staff, who identified a large number of non-conformances when measuring this process.

General conclusions regarding the implementation of this step

There was a consensus of opinion that it was absolutely crucial to recognize the efforts of those who contributed to the quality improvement process at all levels within the organization. The way in which this step was implemented took account of local opinion and tailored the approach to meet this. This was an important part of the success of this step, as the efforts of recognition were accepted by staff as genuine and sincere, rather than a lot of management 'hype'. It was also an important step in changing the culture of the organization to one that visibly valued the efforts of its staff.

The initial eight steps for planning and implementing the quality improvement process using the Crosby approach have now been outlined and illustrated by the practical actions necessary to effect these as taken by the quality improvement team in the case study. As identified earlier, the term 'steps' is somewhat of a misnomer, as they need to be co-ordinated in conjunction with each other. This process will now be explored.

CO-ORDINATION AND PLANNING OF THE FIRST EIGHT STEPS OF THE QUALITY IMPROVEMENT PROCESS

The above eight steps took the QIT 18 months to plan and partially implement. There were some difficulties, as outlined under the specific steps, but one of the biggest factors that was underestimated was the importance of synchronizing the introduction of the different steps in an order that enhanced, rather than inhibited, the corporate impact. This can be overcome by drawing up a comprehensive action plan, which considers the timing of different actions in relation to each other. An example of such a plan is shown in Table 7.1.

The rationale for planning steps in this order is based on a number of factors identified in response to difficulties experienced in practice. These are outlined below:

- *Establish management commitment prior to any public declarations of the implementation of the quality improvement process in the area covered by the QIT.* Staff were quick to point out examples of what they perceived as lack of management commitment to the process.
- *Conduct a general awareness exercise prior to commencing educational courses for staff.* Course facilitators were greatly disadvantaged by staff turning up for courses with no idea of why they were there.

- *Ensure staff have attended the appropriate course prior to any involvement in measurement or problem solving activities.* Problems arose when 'new style' problem solving groups fell back on 'old style' methods of subjective arguments and 'finger pointing' due to some members not having the necessary skills and knowledge.
- *Conduct a 'cost of quality' exercise (or similar baseline audit) early on in the implementation process, and repeat at regular intervals.* When funding became scarce, clear facts and figures to demonstrate benefits were needed.
- *Ensure mechanisms for recognizing the efforts of individuals are established in good time.* Staff were critical of the fact the certificates for the courses were not ready prior to completion by the first groups, and that their efforts were not always acknowledged by senior management.
- *Maintain the momentum of the quality improvement process over a sustained period of time.* After 18 months, the QIT experienced difficulty in maintaining the momentum that was present in the beginning. At this point in time, it is advisable to change some of the team members and re-launch the QIT using the format of the initial 'start-up' day. It was acknowledged that guidance from an experienced facilitator would be extremely beneficial, as many team members felt they had lost direction. A key objective for this day is to produce an action plan for the 14 steps for the following year. At this time, it is appropriate to consider the other steps, which are designed to be introduced at a later stage in the Quality Improvement Process. These are outlined below.

STEP 10: GOAL SETTING

Purpose: To turn pledges and commitments into action by encouraging individuals to establish improvement goals for themselves and their groups.

The need for this step became more apparent following the use of the cost of quality tool, widespread use of measurement and the introduction of the corrective action system. These steps identified areas for improvement, but there was a need to set goals against which progress could be measured. In some areas, in spite of deficiencies identified, nothing further

Table 7.1 Implementation plan for the first year of the quality improvement process

Step no.	Action	Jan	Feb	Mar	Apr	May	Jun	Jul	Aug	Sep	Oct	Nov
Education	QIT complete QES course	X	–X									
	QWG pilot complete	X	–X									
	QES for QIT nominees			X	–	–X						
	QWG facilitator training					X						
	QWG trainers commence course					X						
	QES instructors interviewed			X								
	QES instructors trained			X	–X							
	QES instructors commence					X						
Commitment	Acting UGM 2-day course		X									
	Acting UGM QES			X	–X							
	QIT complete QES	X	–	X								
	Managers mentor QES students			X	–	–	X					
	Quality policy written	X	–	X								
Measurement	Personal measurement	X	–	–	–	–	–	–	–	–	–	–
	QES course members measure		X	–	–	–	–	–	–	–	–	–
	Educate staff re. measurement		X	–	–	–	–	–	–	–	–	–
	Measurement to start in all areas				X	–	–	–	–	–	–	–
Awareness	Collate data collected				X	–	–	–	–	–	–	–
	Feedback results				X	–	–	–	–	–	–	–
	QIT to monitor measurement				X	–	–	–	–	–	–	–
	Prepare information leaflet	X	–X									
	Final draft of leaflet		X									
	Printing of leaflet		X									
	Awareness week planning	X	–X									
	Awareness week		X									
	Poster campaign	X	–	–	–	–	–	–	–	–	–	–
	'Quality' notice board	X	–	–	–	–	–	–	–	–	–	–

Category	Activity	Timeline
Recognition	QIT members report survey results	X
	Criteria for recognition awards	X
	Identify staff for awards	X
	Identify costs	X (Training) ----- X
	Awards presentations	X -----
	Personal recognition from QIT	X ----- X -----
	Photographs of QES/QWG groups	X -----
	Record of QES/QWG 'Roll of Honour'	X ----- X -----
Corrective action	Problem-solving groups identified and measurement commenced	X -----
	Report to QIT	X -----
	Keep register of problems	X ----- X
	Establish CATs to resolve persistant problems	X 18th ----- 18th -----
	Corrective action 'start up' with other QITs	X ----- 22nd April ----- X
Cost of quality	Baseline COQ	X --------------- X
	COQ	X
	Feedback COQ	X
QIT	Formed	Nov. '90
	Start-up day	Nov. '90
	Nominate step sponsors	Nov. '90
	Planning steps	X ----------- X
	'Quality' notice board	X
	Expand QIT ×3 new members	X
	Allocate staff groups to members	X --- X --- X
	Plan awareness week/booklet	X --- X -----
	Nominate QWG Trainers	X
	Educate QIT on QWG	X ----- X
	Further encouragement of audit	X -----
	Further encouragement of measurement	X -----
	Discuss CATs	X -----

CAT, corrective action team; COQ, cost of quality; QIT, Quality Improvement Team; QES, Individual Educaiton Course; QWG, Work Group Education Course; UGM, Unit General Manager.

happened after measurement was completed. Goal setting is required to provide staff with a target, which can be reached through the application of tools and techniques from other steps.

STEPS 7 AND 9: ZERO DEFECTS PLANNING AND ZERO DEFECTS DAY

Purpose, step 7: To examine the various activities that must be conducted in preparation for formally launching Zero Defects Day.
Purpose, step 9: To create an event that will let all employees realize, through a personal experience, that there has been a change.

At the initial QIT educational sessions, concern was expressed over the Crosby anecdotes regarding the baton twirling, brass band parading, balloon releasing events popular with American companies using this approach. These steps therefore lay dormant for a considerable amount of time. They were reconsidered after the success of the 'follow-up' days for course participants, and the poster presentations in the 'Recognition' event. Apart from the advantages of these events in recognizing those who participated, they were also an extremely beneficial way of demonstrating to staff who were still waiting to attend the courses (and those sceptical of the whole approach) the scale of improvements that had arisen as a result of the quality improvement process. Without these, many of the projects would never have been heard about by large groups within the organization. These events also rejuvenated many flagging projects when staff appreciated what had been achieved by many of their peers, and the advice and support offered by these individuals was a far greater motivating force than any management pressure could ever achieve. Although the term 'zero defects day' was confined to the archives, there was an acknowledgement for the need of some kind of event that fulfilled the same purpose.

Step 7 (zero defects planning) was important because an inappropriate or badly planned range of activities could potentially do more harm than good. It was established early on in the quality improvement process that any activity or individual linked directly with the implementation was scrutinized closely by all for evidence of 'Quality'.

STEP 11: ERROR CAUSE REMOVAL

Purpose: To give the individual employee a method of communicating to management the situations that make it difficult to meet the pledge to improve.

This was another step that was regarded initially as an unnecessary bureaucratic venture by the QIT and disregarded in the initial stages of implementation. At this time, problems were commonly being identified through the training courses, and the corrective action system ensured these were dealt with. As time progressed, two major problems of using these methods only were identified.

First, the problems being identified and resolved tended to be on a small scale, of the kind that could be resolved within a discipline or department. These were extremely important but there was a notable lack of the organization-wide problems that we all knew intuitively existed (e.g. the inability of the portering and pharmacy service to meet demand, lack of car parking space, waiting list length and times, and so on). As a result, there was a noted absence of corrective action teams at a senior level, and a paucity of success stories in comparison to those arising from lower down the organization.

The second problem was that once the educational courses stopped there was no method to enable staff to refer problems to the quality improvement team. The corrective action system is designed to involve staff in solving work problems for processes that they can influence. Staff identified numerous 'hassles' in their daily work, which were not appropriate for them to feed into this system as they were not involved personally in the specific process that was creating the difficulty.

The error cause removal system is designed to address these problems. It involves the completion of a simple form, which states 'The following situation is making it difficult to do my job because . . .' or 'The following idea could improve the quality of service in the hospital . . .'

This is then sent to the Error Cause Removal Step Sponsor on the QIT, who initiates the series of events necessary to resolve these. This enables every individual within the organization to raise problems that will be directed to the appropriate individuals who can effect a solution.

Major reservations were expressed on the ability of the QIT

to deal with the potential workload of such a system. A visit to an industrial company 10 years into the quality improvement process showed one team dealing with up to 100 suggestions in one week, and a requirement that all slips received were acknowledged and action arising cited to the initiator within 48 hours. Key factors identified in achieving these requirements were: (i) commitment from senior management (i.e. they allocated time and resources to make the system work); and (ii) the effective establishment of the other steps in creating the culture where such a system can work.

Parallels were drawn with the 'Suggestions box' initiative that had been tried in a number of areas with limited impact. Under the traditional management approach, two things would typically happen if such a system was introduced without the other 13 steps identified by Crosby to support it. One option is that nothing would happen, because staff will not use a system in which they have no confidence. The other is that a few staff will try the system to see what happens. On receiving the forms, the absence of a clearly thought out method for dealing with them leads to two scenarios. One is a defensive exercise to identify either the initiator of the form to argue that no such problem really exists; the other approach is characterized by the manager acknowledging the problem and seeking out the individual who they perceive is responsible for it arising in the first place. Both send negative messages to staff and preclude the use of such systems.

The introduction of error cause removal is the final step in the jigsaw in the quality improvement process. For it to work effectively, the other steps must be firmly in place. When working effectively it offers something no other quality initiative can – the ability of every employee to access the quality improvement system, with the knowledge that appropriate actions will be taken to resolve the problem.

STEP 13: QUALITY COUNCILS

Purpose: To bring together the appropriate people to share quality management information on a regular basis.

Crosby cites the need for individuals with expertise in the quality improvement process to meet regularly to review the approach and generate new ideas. He notes the contribution many former QIT members can make as a result of their experience. In practice, this step was never implemented because in the initial stages, all those with quality management information were heavily involved in the implementation process.

STEP 14: DO IT ALL OVER AGAIN

Purpose: To emphasize that the quality improvement process is continuous.

This step is self-explanatory, but none the less essential. It was important that the quality improvement team created a new action plan on a yearly basis to develop previous work, and maintained the momentum of the quality improvement process. In a rapidly changing sociological/political/economic climate, the requirements of the service are in a constant state of flux, and therefore in need of continual review. From this perspective, the quality improvement process is never-ending. This fact differentiates this approach from that of other 'initiatives' or 'flavour of the month' approaches to managing quality – it is not a project or a programme, but a never ending process.

GENERAL OBSERVATIONS AND KEY LEARNING POINTS FROM THE CASE STUDY

As a result of close involvement in the implementation of the quality improvement process, the following observations are made, based on a personal perspective of the impact of introducing such an approach into a hospital environment.

There are several important factors to consider when reaching conclusions for this specific approach. First, although the framework adopted followed the Crosby 14-step process, this was somewhat anachronistically applied, which undoubtedly created many difficulties. There is a clear recommendation that the whole process should start at the top of the organization and be cascaded down. In practice, a major management restructuring several months into the process meant this did not occur. This posed difficulties for the QIT in the case study, predominantly in the form of lack of clear direction from the steering committee, the constitution of which also changed several months into the process. This meant that systems such as corrective action and error cause removal were not ready at the point which the QIT needed to begin to use them.

The second deviation from the Crosby approach occurred in the use of their educational courses. In this QIT only three out of the eventual 13 members attended the quality improvement course '*à la* Crosby' to prepare them for their role in the implementation process. Approximately 40 staff attended the 'individual' educational course and 120 attended the work group course, at which point the external funding for the pilot site ceased. The percentages in the other QITs were significantly lower than these. It is impossible to draw specific conclusions about the overall impact of educational materials, since two of the key implementation methods were never realized.

It also raises a sombre message about securing adequate funding at the outset of the implementation process. In the case study, the loss of funding created a serious dip in morale for both the team and the course facilitators. It occurred when many of the initial hurdles had been overcome, and benefits were just starting to be realized. What was encouraging, was that the team were sufficiently convinced of the benefits of this approach to resolve to continue, and explore ways of circumnavigating the funding difficulties. This would have been inconceivable 18 months previously, in terms of both commitment to the approach, and the knowledge base of staff.

Key learning points for particular steps are outlined in the text. Although these are derived from the use of the Crosby approach to TQM, many can be extended to the wide range of approaches outlined at the beginning of this chapter.

The need for an overall implementation framework

It is common for those charged with the task of implementing TQM within an organization to feel overwhelmed in regard to the enormity of the scale of the process. A major problem identified in the case study was that lots of texts explore TQM concepts, but very few give definitive ideas on how to implement these into a health care setting. There is a danger of falling into the 'paralysis by analysis' trap in the initial stages of implementation as a result. In our experience, this was typified by long debates over terminology and 'refining' some of the tools and techniques prior to using them.

The major advantage of creating a structure for implementation, be it the 14 steps or another framework, is that it offers those with the responsibility of introducing TQM a clear path to follow. In the QIT in the case study, this proved to be invaluable in focusing the thoughts of members on actions, rather than philosophical debates.

It is strongly recommended that, whatever framework is adopted, the best course of action is to begin it and, if necessary, modify the approach whilst going along. In the early states of the project there was strong pressure to cut out certain aspects and add in others. The key lesson learned in our attempts to customize the approach is not to take out any of the 'bricks' before being clear on why they are there. For example, prior to understanding enough about the process there were suggestions that some of the steps (notably corrective action and error cause removal) were unnecessary and could be dropped. It was not until we were much further into the process that the importance of these was recognized, and this then necessitated a hasty implementation, after a break in the continuity of implementation.

It is important to incorporate a local flavour to the approach and, in practice, we found this was best managed at QIT level rather than further up the organization. There was a marked difference in teams' views on steps such as recognition, based on their local knowledge.

The need for a comprehensive educational programme

In our experience, the educational step, once cascaded throughout the hospital, was an essential factor in generating the desired cultural change.

One problem was the tendency for managers to make assumptions of the ability of their staff to understand tools and techniques. In practice, many of these staff used these tools far more than the managers, as they found them a useful method of identifying and resolving problems in a new way.

Time spent on piloting and modifying courses, training local facilitators to a high standard and on staff education reaped dividends. Attempts to cut costs by modifying this step inevitably cause problems later on.

The need to evaluate the TQM approach

Faced with a project of this scale, methods for formal evaluation may fall low on the list of priorities. The difficulty arises when funding is restricted and objective measures of improvement would prove beneficial. Evaluating such a sizable project, and attempting to control the myriad of variables, is something that defies the bounds of a traditional clinically controlled trial. Faced with all these pressures, the offers from external sources to help in the evaluation process can appear extremely inviting. Based on our experiences, we recommend caution in adopting these offers without careful consideration of the following factors.

First, establish the motives for the offer, which may not always be explicit in the initial contact. Some of the 'surveys' that were circulated to us promising feedback on various approaches were in fact generated from consultancy firms with an interest in TQM. Apart from the danger of bias in such studies, it is worth considering that information supplied is likely to be far more lucrative to the recipient than any subsequent feedback to those who partook in the initial questionnaire.

Second, it is worth critiquing the research design to be used, and the amount of time and effort required by local staff prior to becoming involved in external evaluations. Some of us were rather disconcerted at the use of what was, quite clearly, pre-edited notes being taken throughout personal interviews in one study, rather than tape recording or writing out the interview verbatum. If staff are to be released for such interviews, it is important that a valid and reliable tool is used to make participation worthwhile. Another difficulty can arise if researchers are travelling considerable distances. In one instance this led to a request for a large number of a 'representative cross-section' of staff to be interviewed in one day. Given the clinical commitments of the majority of staff, this was very difficult to organize and, in retrospect, the use of staff who *could* attend, rather than those who *should* attend, did not give a representative sample group.

The timing and appropriateness of interview schedules or questionnaires used by researchers is also worth reviewing. In one study it was not apparent until after staff had been exposed to questioning that the researchers were seeking staff views on benefits seen as a result of using the Crosby method. Many of the staff interviewed had only very recently become involved in the TQM project, many had not completed the relevant courses and the QITs had only recently been formed. It was therefore inappropriate for staff to be expected to contribute valid material at this stage, as it was too early for any objective benefits to be seen.

Several advantages and disadvantages were observed whilst implementing the quality improvement process. These were as follows.

Advantage – breaking down professional and hierarchical barriers. The multidisciplinary nature of the quality improvement team did much to improve communication and understanding between the different disciplines. This was particularly noted as part of the educational courses throughout all levels of the organization, where staff gained insight into the roles and responsibilities of colleagues, often for the first time. This undoubtedly helped to break down barriers, as staff tended to become more sympathetic to the difficulties of other groups and endeavoured to help them solve their work problems.

Advantage – beginning the process of changing from a 'finger-pointing' culture. The major advantage in adopting the tools and techniques in this approach was that it focused the staff's attention on aspects of the work process where requirements were not being met (or were not established) rather than on the traditional approach of blaming errors on specific individuals. This process of 'de-personalizing' problems proved a useful method of reducing the conflict when staff attempted to resolve them.

Advantage – providing a 'common language' for communicating about quality. This original claim by those advocating the Crosby approach was met with some scepticism by many staff. However, as more staff undertook the course, it was noticeable how the phrases initially criticized as 'jargon' had slipped into the general vocabulary. The advantage of phrases like 'non-conformance', 'requirements', etc. is that, once staff have been educated as to their meaning, they are uniformly understood by all. The widespread use of the same tools (such as the process model worksheet and measurement charts) by all departments and professional groups also provided a valuable uniform approach to addressing problems.

In an area such as health care that is littered with confusing terminology, it is interesting the amount of resistance there is to 'non-health' terminology. The important lesson learned was that the phrase was less important than the universal understanding of that phrase. For example, one would not refuse to use 'computerized axial tomography purely because the name of the tool is complicated. The important thing is to understand what the machine is used for. The name may be shortened to 'CAT scan', as this is more 'user-friendly', but this does not detract from the staff's understanding of its purpose. So it is for terms such as 'zero defects'. The important factor is in the benefit of the tool, rather than the phrase itself. This can be changed to suit local needs if necessary, but it would be foolhardy to discard a useful tool on the basis of its name alone.

Advantage – providing a systematic approach for managing quality. This approach offered an umbrella under which to pull all of the different quality initiatives and ensure they were managed in a systematic way. This is the big advantage of using the quality improvement process, as its ability to encompass all the activities and individuals within an organization offers far-reaching benefits for all customers and suppliers.

Disadvantage – threat of change. The implementation of the quality improvement process can prove enormously threatening because it implies criticism of traditional management methods. The implementation structure requires those most sensitive to these criticisms to throw their full weight behind the changes. The whole process of empowering staff can also be interpreted as an undermining of the 'position power' of the hierarchical line manager, and it is a power some are unhappy to relinquish. It can therefore prove an uncomfortable process for many individuals.

Disadvantage – raising customer expectations. 'Going public' on the organizational commitment to TQM undoubtedly raised the expectations of internal and external customers. This can be a disadvantage if the mechanisms are not in place to ensure they can be met.

Disavantage – substantial initial investment before returns are realized. All the authors in this field emphasize that TQM is a long-term investment. Full implementation can take up to 5 years, and the process must be on-going if the benefits are to be sustained. Those who view this as a short-term initiative and expect immediate results will be disappointed. In consequence, a significant initial financial investment is required, with no visible financial returns for several years.

CONCLUSIONS REGARDING THE USE OF THE CROSBY METHOD OF TOTAL QUALITY MANAGEMENT

It has been stated that our intention was not to indulge in a war of armchair theory, advocating the finer philosophical points of one approach to TQM over another. This would be unfair in the absence of 'hands-on' experience of more than one approach. For this reason, conclusions can only be drawn on the Crosby approach.

From a purely practical perspective, as a result of using this method, we believe it to be a comprehensive system that is flexible enough to be adapted for use in hospitals. However, the use of expertise of committed personnel from within the hospital is a key factor in adapting it to a health care environment.

On re-reading the works of other leaders in this field (notably Deming, Juran, Koch and Shaw) there are common themes:

- The need for management commitment and leadership.
- The need to empower the workers.
- The need to establish clear requirements or specifications, and meet these every time.
- The value of breaking down the work process into a number of identifiable steps and using the increased understanding gained during the process to find and eliminate quality problems.
- Focusing on the prevention of problems or errors.
- Utilizing statistical techniques.
- Recognition that quality is a never-ending process.

These similarities (and other clear differences) can be confusing to those attempting to select one (or a combination of several) systems for implementation. A framework for evaluating and selecting a quality improvement process has been developed by Fine (1986), based on three dimensions:

- *Decision rules and decision tools.* This examines the three decision tools for quality management: (i) cost of quality; (ii) direct (physical) measures of quality; and (iii) revenue and cost of quality and their value in specific type of organizations.
- *Managerial style.* This is defined as 'the philosophy behind the management of the human resources of the firm'. In essence, this is divided into authoritarian and participative styles. It explores the underlying management theories of Deming, Crosby and Juran, and their adaptability under differing organizational styles of management.
- *The management of the transition to TQM.* This examines theoretical basis of the specific approach by referring to the theories of organizational change.

Using the above framework to analyse the Crosby approach, its creators drew the following conclusions.

First, that the Crosby approach presents a management style that is predominantly authoritarian but has some participative elements. All employees are told what is expected of them, but they have input into identifying and solving problems. Because of this, the Crosby process can accommodate a range of management styles.

Second, that the Crosby process could be viewed as 'a classic example of how to manage transition' (Bridge, 1984). The 14-step programme meets almost every criterion set by Beckhard and Harris (1977) for managing complex changes in organizations.

The purpose of utilizing this framework is to allow the selection of an approach that best meets the specific individualized need of the organization. For example, it has been observed that organizations that are predominantly authoritarian may have difficulty in adopting the managerial style advocated in some of the TQM approaches.

In conclusion, by far the most important factor in adopting this whole process is the realization by senior management that TQM is worthwhile, and their decision to commit themselves to

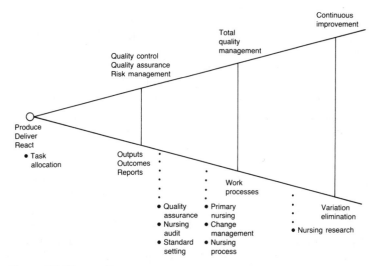

Figure 7.3 The quality spectrum.

adopting its principles. Once this has been decided, the selection of the methods used becomes an essential, but nevertheless academic, argument on which specific approach (or the decision to use an eclectic model) offers the best method for their organization.

FINAL SUMMARY AND CONCLUSIONS

Following the theme of 'making quality happen', some general observations have been made:

- That standard-setting can be an extremely useful tool for improving quality but, unless standards are audited, their full potential is not realized.
- That audit is an important part in establishing an understanding of strong and weak areas in clinical practice, but that without a framework for implementation and monitoring there is a danger of developing uncoordinated, unreliable tools. The full potential is therefore not realized.
- That quality assurance offers a number of validated tools and a logical framework for applying these tools. However, without a fundamental understanding of how to manage change there is a danger that quality assurance becomes a

'paperchase' that fails to have any impact on improving clinical nursing practice; its full potential is therefore never realized.

- That effective management of change in nursing, through the use of the tools outlined above, enables the development and improvement in clinical practice that will ultimately benefit the patient. Focusing narrowly on the nursing profession excludes other groups that have the ability to contribute to clinical practice, as their full potential is never realized.

This poses the question as to where such initiatives rest, in relation both to each other and to the concept of 'making quality happen'. The relationship is best demonstrated by examining the model in Figure 7.3 (Creative Factory Inc. 1992).

The quality spectrum starts with the traditional notion that quality will just 'happen on its own', and does not need to be managed. This is demonstrated by the 'produce/deliver/react' response to quality management. Hence the approach is reactive and uncoordinated.

The second phase involves the widening of the spectrum to incorporate quality control, quality assurance and risk management. This occurs when it is realized that 'quality' may be a definable commodity and attempts are made to measure this. Such approaches focus on the output or the outcome of the work process, and provide an indication of how the processes are functioning. This focus on outcome does not indicate *why* such an outcome is achieved, and is also retrospective.

The third phase involves further expansion of the spectrum to include total quality management. This approach focuses on understanding the whole work process, understanding why and how certain outcomes are achieved and on instigating a process of improvement.

The final phase indicated on the spectrum adds a further dimension – that of continuous improvement. This phase examines and monitors the causes of variation in the work processes and provides the tools and techniques for the accurate prediction and control of the outcome by manipulating the variables that influence the process.

The spectrum does not show a discrete end to these phases, as quality management is a new art that is rapidly developing and extending.

The quality spectrum shown in Figure 7.3 also indicates the relative positions of some of the nursing initiatives taken to improve quality within this book. The starting point on the spectrum can be illustrated by the 'task allocated' approach to care delivery. Nursing standard-setting and nursing audit focus predominantly on nursing outcomes. They are shown slightly to the right of this line on the spectrum, as it is acknowledged these tools can also be used to analyse the nursing process as well as outcomes.

The nursing process itself, along with the movement towards Primary Nursing, are seen further along the spectrum towards total quality management. Both of these initiatives are an attempt to understand and improve the process of nursing.

Nursing research is shown as moving towards continuous improvement by reducing variation elimination. Through research, the nursing profession can identify the most effective methods for improving and organizing care.

It can be seen from the spectrum that there is the potential for moving quality management through these phases as a basis for improving the quality of care. It can also be appreciated, from both the spectrum, and from examples throughout the book, that the quality of nursing care is dependent on a myriad of variables, some of which fall outside the sphere of influence of nurses. This creates a need to examine the concept of quality within the wider context of the organization. It is this recognition, together with the knowledge and determination to take action to address the whole issue of quality management in nursing, that is the first, fundamental step towards 'making quality happen'.

REFERENCES

Audit Commission (Stationery Office) (1991) *Lying in Wait: The use of medical beds in acute hospitals*, Audit Commission, London.

Beckhard, R. and Harris R.T. (1977) *Organizational Transitions: Managing complex change*, Addison Wesley, Reading, Massachusetts.

Bendell T. (1990) *The Quality Gurus*, Department Of Trade and Industry/Barnes and Humby Ltd, Nottingham.

Berwick, D.M., Enthoven, A. and Bunker J.P. (1992a) Quality management in the N.H.S: the doctor's role – I. *British Medical Journal*, **304**, 235–9.

Berwick, D.M., Enthoven, A. and Bunker J.P. (1992b) Quality management in the N.H.S: the doctor's role – II *British Medical Journal*, **304**: 304–8.

Bridge, D.E. (1984) *The Role of Managerial Accounting in Quality Improvement Programmes*. MIT Master's Thesis, Sloan School of Management.

Claus, L.M. (1991) Total quality management: A healthcare application *Total Quality Management*, **2** (2), 131–48.

Creative Factory Inc. (1992) Philip Crosby Associates Inc., 3260 University Boulevard, Po Box 6006, Winter Park, Florida.

Crosby, P.B. (1979) *Quality is Free*, McGraw-Hill Book Co., New York.

Crosby, P.B. (1988) *The Eternally Successful Organisation: The art of corporate wellness*, McGraw-Hill Book Co., New York.

Crosby, P.B. (1991) *Quality Improvement Process Management College* (course material), The Creative Factory Inc., Florida.

Cullen, J. and Hollingham (1987) *Implementing Total Quality*, I.F.S. (Publications) Ltd, London.

Fine, C.H. and Bridge, D.H. (1987) *Quest for Quality: Managing the Total System*. Institute of Industrial Engineers, Industrial Engineering and Management Press, New York.

Gitlow, H.S. and Gitlow, S.J. (1987) *The Deming Guide To Quality and Competitive Position*. Prentice-Hall Inc, Englewood Cliffs, New Jersey.

Hibbs, P. (1988) *Pressure Area Care for the City and Hackney Health Authority*, City and Hackney Health Authority, West Smithfield, London.

Mortiboys, R.J. (1990) *Leadership and Total Quality Management: A Guide for Chief Executives*. Department of Trade and Industry/Moore and Matthes Group Ltd, London.

Oberle, J. (1990) Quality gurus the men and their message. *Training*, **January**, 47–52.

Scherkenbach, W.W. (1986) *The Deming Route to Quality and Productivity: Road Maps and Road Blocks*, Mercury Press/Fairchild Publications, Rockville, Maryland.

Index

Page numbers appearing in **bold** refer to figures and page numbers appearing in *italic* refer to tables.